T0191465

A PRACTICAL GUIDE TO
EQUINE RADIOGRAPHY

A PRACTICAL GUIDE TO EQUINE RADIOGRAPHY

Gabriel Manso Díaz

Javier López San Román

Renate Weller

Photography: Javier Sanz Dueñas

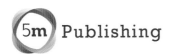

5m Publishing

First published 2018

Reprinted 2021

Published by
5M Publishing Ltd,
Benchmark House,
8 Smithy Wood Drive,
Sheffield, S35 1QN, UK
Tel: +44 (0) 1234 81 81 80
www.5mpublishing.com

A Catalogue record for this book is available from the British Library

ISBN 9781789180145

Book layout by Keystroke, Neville Lodge, Tettenhall, Wolverhampton
Printed by Replika Press Pvt Ltd, India
Photos by Javier Sanz Dueñas

CONTENTS

LIST OF FIGURES AND TABLES

ABOUT THE AUTHORS

Javier López-Sanromán – DVM, PhD, Dipl ECVS
Javier graduated from Complutense University of Madrid (UCM) in Spain, and subsequently obtained a PhD in equine arthroscopy. He is also Diplomate of the European College of Veterinary Surgeons. He is Associate Professor in Equine Surgery at the Department of Animal Medicine and Surgery of the UCM where he currently is the Head of the Large Animal Clinic of the Veterinary Teaching Hospital. He is heavily involved in teaching undergraduate veterinary students (general surgery, equine medicine and surgery, and lameness diagnosis) and postgraduate students (sedation and analgesia in the equine patient). His research interests include equine surgical diseases, antibiotic therapies, sedation and analgesia and gait analysis.

Gabriel Manso-Díaz – DVM, MSc, PhD, MRCVS
Gabriel graduated from the Complutense University of Madrid (UCM) in Spain, and then completed a Master in Research in Veterinary Sciences. After this, he did a PhD on comparison of advanced imaging modalities in the diagnosis of head disorders in the horse. Gabriel splits his time between clinical work in veterinary diagnostic imaging and clinical research, with a particular emphasis on equine head, spinal and abdominal imaging. He currently works at the Diagnostic Imaging Department of the Veterinary Teaching Hospital of the UCM and at the Equine Diagnostic Imaging Department at the Royal Veterinary College in London, UK.

Renate Weller – Drvetmed, PhD, MScVetEd, FHEA, NTF, Dipl. ACVSMR, Dipl ECVSMR, AssocECVDI, MRCVS
After graduating from the University of Munich in Germany, Renate spent a year in the US before she returned to Germany to work in equine practice. She then became a Senior Clinical Research Scholar in Large Animal Diagnostic Imaging at the Royal Veterinary College (RVC) in London, UK. After this, she joined the Institute of Veterinary Anatomy in Munich, where she completed her Dr.Vet.Med. thesis on comparison of different imaging modalities in the diagnosis of head disorders in the horse. Following this, she spent two years in the US before returning to the RVC to do a PhD in the Structure and Motion Laboratory investigating the effect of conformation on locomotor biomechanics in the horse. Since 2005 Renate has been employed at the RVC dividing her time between clinical work in Large Animal Diagnostic Imaging and research in imaging, locomotor biomechanics and veterinary education.

CHAPTER 1

How to get the most from your X-ray system

What determines the success of a diagnostic imaging procedure?

A diagnostic imaging procedure is considered successful if it aids in getting the correct diagnosis. This is influenced by several factors – apart from the size and type of lesion which cannot be influenced by the investigator: it includes the correct choice of modality, the quality of the image and the expertise of the person interpreting the images.

Correct choice of modality: when does taking radiographs make sense?

Radiographs are indicated to:

- confirm a clinically suspected diagnosis
- assess the severity of a disease
- exclude other pathological conditions
- assist in surgery planning
- monitor the progress of disease.

Please bear in mind the following.

- No imaging technique can replace the clinical examination! Radiographic findings do not indicate pain!
- The clinical findings need to guide radiography, e.g. a wound, swelling or positive regional analgesia need to point to an area.

- Using imaging as a 'fishing exercise' is not a good idea, since most changes observed on images may or may not be of clinical significance and their clinical meaning can only be appreciated in conjunction with the clinical findings.
- An exception is pre-purchase and pre-sales radiographs, where an attempt is made to use radiography as a predictor for future soundness and performance.

Basic principles of the underlying physics of radiographs

Understanding how radiographs are produced and what radiographs can show/not show will help to make the correct decision as to their use.

How are X-rays produced?

- X-rays are electromagnetic waves from the high-energy end of the electromagnetic spectrum (visible light or radio waves are part of the same spectrum, but of lower energy and different wave length).
- X-rays are produced when fast-moving electrons collide with matter. This happens in an X-ray tube that houses a cathode and an anode. By heating up the cathode, a cloud of electrons (negatively charged particles) is

produced, which are accelerated by applying a current to the system until they hit the positive anode at high speed.

- The higher the temperature of the cathode, the more electrons are produced; this is related to the mAs (milliampere seconds) settings of the X-ray machine.
- The higher the speed of the electrons, the higher the penetrating power of the resulting X-rays. This is controlled by the kVp settings of the X-ray machine.
- X-rays radiate from the source in straight lines in all directions. For medical purposes, only a small cone of the X-rays, the primary beam, is used.
- The size of the primary beam is set by adjusting the window through which X-rays can leave the housing of the X-ray generator. This is called collimation and is an essential radiation protection mechanism, but also optimizes image quality by reducing scatter.
- The intensity of the X-ray beam is inversely proportional to the square of the distance from the source ('inverse square law'). This is obviously important for radiation safety consideration and has to be taken into account when adjusting exposure settings. Figure 1.1 illustrates this effect.

How do X-rays interact with matter?

- When X-rays hit matter, they can either penetrate the material or get absorbed by it. The main underlying principles on an atomic level are called the Compton and the photoelectric effect. The Compton effect is less desirable since it is responsible for scatter radiation that degrades image quality.
- The degree of absorption of the X-rays by material is determined by the thickness and the radiodensity of the absorber.
- The radiodensity depends on the physical density and the atomic number of the material, e.g. lead has a very high atomic number which allows complete absorption of X-rays with only a few millimetres of material. This is the reason why, for example, lead is used for shielding purposes, e.g. in protective clothing. The same effect can be achieved with material of lower atomic number by increasing its thickness, e.g. a 20 cm brick wall.
- The body is composed of materials of different radiodensities and thickness, hence X-rays are absorbed differentially. For example, bone has a higher radiodensity and hence absorbs more X-rays than soft tissue, hence bone appears whiter on the resulting image

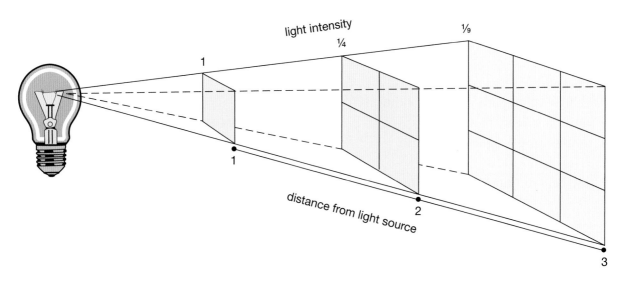

Figure 1.1 This figure illustrates the effect of distance on X-ray intensity, 'inverse square law'. The intensity of the X-ray beam is inversely proportional to the square of the distance from the source. This is obviously important for radiation safety consideration and must be taken into account when adjusting exposure settings.

than soft tissues. This provides the basis for the image contrast that allows differentiation between structures on radiographs.

How are X-rays registered and how is that transformed into an image?

- While the way X-rays are generated has not changed much, the way they are detected has undergone considerable changes in the last few years.
- Conventionally, X-rays are detected using photographic film in combination with intensifying screens. After exposure, the film needs developing in a similar process to film-based photography to produce the final radiograph.
- Computed radiography (CR) systems still require the use of cassettes and a processor. A phosphor-coated plate in the cassette absorbs X-rays and stores them as energy. The stored energy is released as visible light after stimulation of the atoms on the phosphor plate with a laser beam in the processor. The light is registered and converted into a digital signal. After erasing the imaging plate, it can then be reused.
- In digital radiography (DR) systems, the image is displayed directly on a screen without the necessity of processing a plate.

You will find more information on this in Chapter 2.

What can radiographs show?

- Radiographs can show changes in tissue density, shape, size, outline and position of structures.
- Radiographs in the horse are primarily used to assess bones but can also provide information about soft tissues.

When do we see changes in bone on radiographs?

- Bone is a dynamic tissue and undergoes constant changes in response to the stress it is put under (Wolff's law). This results in changes in bone density, size, shape and outline which can be a physiological process but also changes with pathology. A good example of physiological adaptation of bone to increased stress turning into a pathological process is the changes observed in the skeletal system of racehorses, for example in the third carpal bone.
- A 30–50% change in mineralization of a bone is required until it can be visualized on radiographs. This makes radiographs a relatively insensitive tool to detect these changes and they often indicate advanced pathology.
- Once radiographic abnormalities have developed they can persist for a long time without being clinically significant; a good example of this is the presence of osteophytes indicating joint osteoarthritis without any clinical signs.

How does an increase in bone production appear on radiographs?

New bone production appears as opacity on radiographs and can be classified according to the location:

- Enthesophytes: focal, distinct new bone formation at attachment site of ligaments, tendons and joint capsules, usually associated with chronic strain at this site.
- Osteophytes: periarticular new bone usually associated with osteoarthritis.
- Sclerosis: a term used for localized new bone formation, usually in response to stress (e.g. subchondral bone sclerosis in osteoarthritis) or when the body is walling off areas, e.g. a sequestrum or bone cyst.
- Periosteal new bone: often caused by trauma but can also be caused by infection.

- Endosteal new bone: most commonly associated with trauma, e.g. fractures, but can also be caused by infection or inflammation.
- Cortical thickening: in response to stress.
- Callus formation: fracture repair.

How does a decrease in bone production appear on radiographs?

Bone resorption results in lysis of bone and appears radiographically as radiolucency. This is most commonly focal in the horse but can also be diffuse.

- Focal lucencies:

  - Changes in bone contour, e.g. flattening of trochlear ridges in cases of osteochondrosis.
  - Well-defined lucencies within bone, e.g. osseous cyst-like lesions.
  - Subchondral bone lucencies, e.g. in osteoarthritis.

- Diffuse lesions:

  - Diffuse bone resorption affecting whole bones is, for example, seen with disuse osteopenia and results in a honeycomb appearance of the bone structure. This is often most easily appreciated in the proximal sesamoid bones or the distal phalanx.
  - Diffuse heterogenous lesions are a radiographic sign of neoplastic processes; however, bone tumours are extremely rare in horses!

What can radiographs tell us about soft tissues?

- Radiographs are not very sensitive when it comes to the assessment of different soft tissue densities: e.g. fluids such as blood or urine have the same radiographic appearance as most other soft tissues (tendons, cartilage, etc.).
- The exception is fat, which appears more radiolucent than other soft tissues, which can, for example, be appreciated in the case of the triangular radiolucency consistent with the patellar fat pad in the stifle or on the dorsal aspect of the carpus. The disappearance of these may indicate pathology of the respective joint.
- Abdominal radiography:

  - The sheer size of an adult horse makes it impossible to get detailed radiographs of the adult abdomen. One exception where abdominal radiographs may be useful is to visualize the presence of sand or enteroliths in the gut.
  - Abdominal radiographs in foals are commonly performed to evaluate the gastrointestinal tract and render diagnostic results similar to small animals.

- Thoracic radiography:

  - This is best performed with a high-output X-ray machine and a grid for scatter reduction, hence is usually only done in hospital settings.
  - It is not very sensitive for most thoracic disease and its usefulness should be considered very carefully in each case, especially since it involves high radiation exposures!

CHAPTER 2

X-ray equipment and radiation safety in equine practice

The equipment needed for equine radiography includes:

- X-ray generator
- registration plates or cassettes to register the image
- stands and holders for equipment: plate holders, generator stands
- positioning aids for horses: blocks, head stand
- anti-scatter grids
- protective equipment:

  - gowns, thyroid protectors, gloves
  - screens
  - monitoring badges

- viewing station
- visual warning aids such as signs or tape if necessary to prevent people walking in on the procedure
- competent horse handler
- Sedation!

X-ray generators

X-ray generators can be divided into portable, mobile and stationary machines. Portable machines are small and lightweight units that can easily be fitted in a car and carried by hand and are commonly used in equine ambulatory practice. Mobile machines are on wheels and can be moved around within a hospital setting. These are often used if no dedicated X-ray room is available and X-ray procedures are performed in rooms where other procedures also take place, for example operating theatres. Stationary units are usually ceiling-mounted units in dedicated X-ray suites.

X-ray generators are categorized based on their output into 'high-output' and 'low-output' generators. Stationary machines are usually high-output generators while portable machines are limited in their output and mobile machines are somewhere between the two. The output capacity of a machine can be found in the technical specification of the equipment and usually also on a sticker on the side of the generator. Both the maximum kVp and the maximum mA should be listed. It is well worth being familiar with these values since it will let the user decide which radiographs are within the capability of the system.

Registration systems: computed versus digital radiography

Recent advancements in diagnostic imaging have seen the replacement of conventional film-screen systems with computed radiography

(CR) or digital radiography (DR) systems and these are now the mainstay systems used in equine practice.

Computerized systems still use cassettes that are then digitized in a laser scanner whereas digital systems use a digital plate that transmits the image directly to a computer for display. CR cassettes need cleaning on a regular basis and erasing if they have not been in use for a while. Both DR and CR systems produce digital images that are manipulated and viewed on a computer. Care should be taken that the spatial and contrast resolution of the viewing screen is not compromising image quality.

CR and DR systems offer a multitude of options during and after image acquisition. Some image quality parameters are specific to the individual system and it is well worth paying attention to those when choosing a system to buy. It is advisable to spend time with an application technician of the specific company where you bought the system and include this time in the purchase price. Application technicians are people trained to have the skills and knowledge to get the best possible quality image out of a system while keeping the exposures to a minimum.

What is considered the best image differs between individuals and also between applications and hence depends on case load but also personal preference. For example, in racehorse practice, subtle changes to bone trabecular pattern might be more important than the ability to appreciate soft tissue changes on radiographs and hence the standard settings of the way the image is acquired, processed and viewed will differ from that of a general riding horse population. Of course, the standard settings can and should be adapted to each individual case.

The world of imaging technology is changing rapidly and it is well worth checking standard procedures regularly; for example, DR plates are becoming more and more sensitive to X-rays and hence exposures can be decreased and areas where it was previously impossible to acquire

diagnostic quality radiographs with portable machines might be now accessible.

Plates come in different sizes. Smaller plates are preferable for the distal limb, whereas larger plates are helpful for the spine, pelvis and thorax. While shoulder and stifle radiographs can be taken with smaller plates, people often find these easier with larger plates.

Grids

Grids can be used to reduce scatter. This is especially an issue in upper body radiographs that require high exposures and where there are lots of soft tissues present. Some users also find them helpful for the navicular bone. Many DR and CR systems have digital grids that make the use of hardware grids redundant and it is well worth testing out if the use of a grid is necessary since grids have the disadvantage that they require an increase in exposure and perfect alignment.

Stands and holders for equipment

It is common in equine practice to hand-hold portable X-ray generators, since it is easy to do and speeds up the procedure. This is not advisable since it leads to an unnecessary increase in radiation exposure to the operator. It also increases the likelihood of movement artefacts, especially with higher exposure radiographs where the time of exposure is longer. There are several stands for X-ray generators on the market (Fig. 2.1). These stands are height adjustable and fold, so can be fitted in a car. If a purpose-made stand is not available, one can also be inventive and use blocks of wood or buckets to position an X-ray generator at the required height.

Plates/cassettes should not be held by hand since this brings the hand very close to the primary beam and also results in unnecessary radiation exposure to the person holding it. Long-handled plate holders should be available so that the person holding the plate can step away as far as possible from the primary

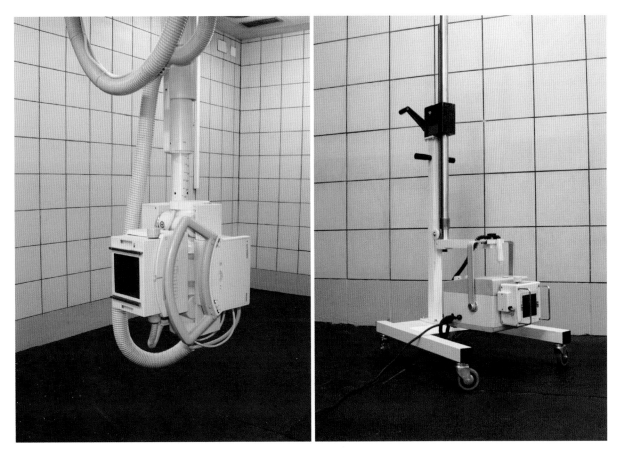

Figure 2.1 On the left there is a ceiling-mounted X-ray generator. On the right, a portable X-ray generator with a purpose-made stand can be observed.

beam. Ideally, they are custom-built for the specific systems; however, should these not be available, one can resort to using a broomstick and duct tape. Shorter handles are helpful for radiographs of the stifle, where longer handles are too cumbersome (and dangerous) to use.

Ceiling-mounted systems allow for using a ceiling-mounted plate holding system, that ideally moves in a synchronized fashion with the X-ray generator and guarantees automatic perfect alignment, facilitating image acquisition of the spine, pelvis and thorax. If such a ceiling-mounted, movable plate holder is not available, one may consider taping plates to an available wall and positioning the horse in front of it accordingly.

Positioning aids for horses

Several blocks are helpful to position the horse's foot. To be able to centre correctly for radiographs of a horse's foot, the foot has to be raised in relation to the X-ray beam since the central X-ray beam is usually not low enough. This can be achieved by putting the horse on blocks. Ideally, both feet are on a block each since this is more comfortable for the horse and hence better tolerated. Assessment of foot conformation should be part of any foot study and for this it is preferable that the feet are equally weight-bearing.

Hickman (also called Oxspring) blocks are blocks that position the horse's foot at a given angle and facilitate oblique views of the navicular bone (see Fig. 4.14). The same views can also be achieved in the weight-bearing horse using a tunnel block (see Fig. 4.13).

Sedation is often advisable in achieving diagnostic radiographs in an acceptable time frame with minimum stress to horse and danger to staff. Sedation-induced ataxia and head dropping can be limited by allowing the horse to rest its head either on a custom-built head-stand or on, for example, a bale of shavings. This not only aids in reducing movement but it also helps to standardize the position of the horse in relation to the X-ray beam; this helps when radiographs of the neck or head have to be repeated due to missing the structure of interest. It also standardizes the neck position, which influences the alignment of the cervical as well as thoracic vertebrae and the width of the interspinous spaces in the back.

Protective equipment

Considering radiation safety is essential when taking radiographs. It is not only a legal requirement but it is now well known that ionizing radiation has no threshold for damage, but that every exposure increases the risk of not only developing cancer but also the occurrence of other diseases, such as strokes and heart attacks. Protective clothing is only part of radiation safety considerations.

Equine radiography is somewhat different to human and small animal radiography, since equine practitioners are allowed to use ionizing radiation in the field in the presence of lay people. Unlike in human and small animal radiography, equine radiography commonly involves the use of a horizontal X-ray beam, and hence the user has to consider very carefully where the beam travels.

Whatever we do, we should always follow the ALARA (As Low As Reasonably Achievable) principle and make sure we keep the radiation exposure to everybody as low as possible while staying safe around the horse.

Make sure that:

1. Only the minimum number of people necessary are involved while having the horse adequately handled. This usually requires a minimum of one and a maximum of three people depending on the type of procedure and the temperament of the horse.

2. The risk of exposing people incidentally is minimized. Put up visual signs such as a sign or tape that prevents people entering your X-ray area. Direct your X-ray beam against a brick wall or if radiographing in a wooden stable, make sure nobody stands or walks behind the stable.

3. People involved in the procedure wear protective clothing, including gown and thyroid protector and gloves if necessary. Remember that protective clothing only protects from scatter radiation, not from primary beam radiation.

4. No human body parts are included in the collimated area.

5. The exposures are kept to the minimum. Since the sensitivity of plates is increasing, this ought to be checked when equipment is upgraded.

6. You know what you are doing! Incompetence may lead to unnecessary repeats of exposures.

Protective clothing comes in different thicknesses (mm lead equivalent) and you need to check with your local authorities to find out what is required. You may also consider whether a gown or a top and skirt are better for your purposes. All protective clothing needs to be checked for cracks and holes in the protective layer on a regular basis by radiographing them. Please take care to store protective clothing correctly by hanging the gowns up for example – do not put them in a crumpled heap in your car!

Other protective equipment may include the use of lead screens which are limited to stationary settings. These are positioned strategically within a room for staff to stand behind during exposure.

Monitoring equipment

Personal monitoring equipment is a legal requirement in most countries for workers who are likely to be exposed to ionizing radiation on a regular basis or doses that may go beyond the legal limit. Personal monitoring equipment consists of lightweight badges that are pinned either under or over protective clothing depending on country-specific regulations. The badges are sent off at regular intervals to be read and a personal radiation log is created. Electronic dosimeters that give an instant reading are also available but are more expensive than badges. There are also dosimeters available that are used to record room exposure.

A book to record exposures is also often required to keep a log of radiation exposures.

Since there are distinct differences between countries, please contact your local authorities to find out about your specific regulations.

CHAPTER 3

Image quality

How do we assess image quality and what can we do to get the best possible image?

Image quality is one of the main parameters that influences the diagnostic success of an imaging procedure. The better an image, the easier lesions can be detected and misinterpretations avoided.

What image parameters characterize a radiograph?

The following parameters all determine image quality and are influenced by our equipment and the way we take and process our images:

- image resolution
- sharpness
- image contrast
- signal-to-noise ratio
- exposures
- distortion and magnification
- artefacts.

Image resolution

- Image resolution quantifies how close structures can be to each other and still be visibly resolved and provides a measure of detail.
- In conventional radiography, it is usually expressed as line pairs/mm (10–15 lp/mm). In CR/DR radiography it is expressed in pixels, similar to what you will be familiar with in photo cameras and smartphones.
- Image resolution is set by the manufacturer and cannot be changed in DR systems; however, in CR systems different plates with different types of resolution are available. While the standard plates are sufficient for most applications, high-resolution plates may be better for looking at fine trabecular detail.
- There are no guidelines in veterinary medicine as to the minimum resolution a system needs to have; however, there are in human medicine and usually the systems on the veterinary market follow those as well.
- Beware of the image resolution of the screen you are viewing your images on. It is pointless having a high-resolution image to start with if you are viewing it on a low-resolution screen.
- Equally, beware of how an image is sent. The default image format in which images are sent is JPG which, as standard, compresses images and this may well result in loss of image quality.

Image sharpness

- Image sharpness describes how well the edges of a structure can be distinguished from other structures or the background. Image sharpness is affected by the equipment but also by the way we take radiographs.

- It is influenced by the following.

  - Focus–film distance (FFD): the bigger, the sharper; try to avoid going below the standard 100 cm FFD. The focus point of a high-output machine is usually marked by a red dot; in portable machines you may assume it is somewhere in the centre.
  - Distance between the object and the X-ray plate: the smaller, the sharper. Make sure you keep your plate as close to the horse as is safely possible. This also minimizes magnification (Fig. 3.1).
  - Movement blur: this can be caused by movement of the horse, the plate or the X-ray generator. The risk of movement blur can be minimized by the following:

  - Using plate and X-ray machine stands rather than hand-holding equipment. This has the added advantage of reducing radiation exposure to yourself and others.
  - Use of a head stand may help steady the whole horse.
  - Adequate sedation; a combination of butorphanol and detomidine or romifidine usually works well.
  - Keeping exposure times as short as possible. This may be challenging for the higher exposure radiographs since small machines are limited in their mA output, hence times must lengthen for higher exposures. As a rule of thumb, try to keep the exposure time under 0.2 s.

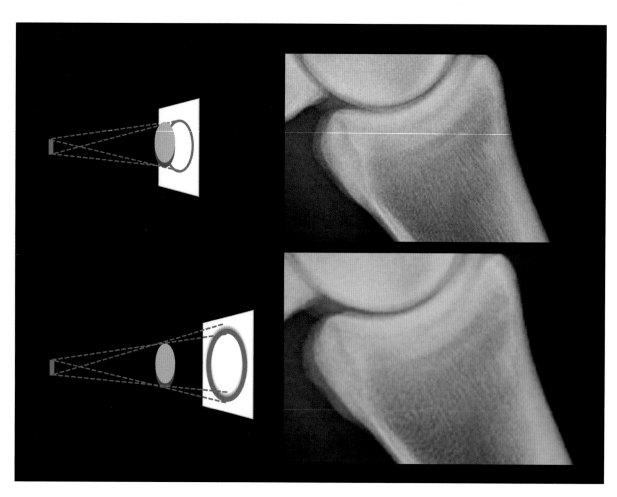

Figure 3.1 This figure illustrates the effect of object–plate distance on image sharpness and magnification. In the image on the top, the plate was close to the fetlock joint on this lateromedial radiograph, compared to the bottom image where there was a distance between the two. The image on the top has sharper edges and is smaller compared to the bottom image.

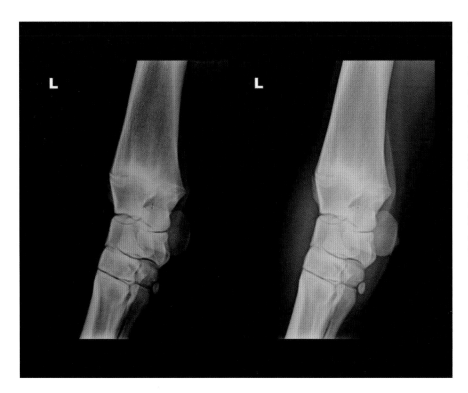

Figure 3.2 This figure shows the same radiograph in different window levels. The image on the right is windowed to highlight the soft tissue envelope, whereas the image on the left shows more bone detail. The ability to change brightness and contrast of a radiograph is a huge benefit of digital images and enhances our ability to assess these.

– Post-processing: many systems have edge enhancement options. Beware that these can also lead to a false impression of sharpness.
– Size of the focal spot: the smaller, the sharper, something to consider when buying a new X-ray machine.
– Poor screen–film contact in conventional radiography.

Image contrast

• Image contrast is the difference in radiodensity that makes an object distinguishable from another structure.
• It is expressed as contrast resolution and is a measure of the grey values. The more 'greys' an image displays, the more structures of different radiodensities it can distinguish.
• The pixel depth (in bits per pixel) is a measurement for contrast resolution (grey value) of the image. For example, a 1-bit image shows only black and white, an 8-bit image shows 256 greys and a 12-bit image, 4096.
• Image contrast depends on:

– Detector: different systems have different contrast and this should be considered when buying a new system
– Object: size and radiodensity; this is obviously out of the control of the operator
– Exposure values: this is a major factor and exposure settings are discussed in detail below
– Image processing: DR and CR systems offer many post-processing and viewing options. You should work with an application technician to get the most out of it
– Image display: make sure your viewing screen has an adequate range of contrast. When you view an image, changing contrast and brightness often enable you to gain additional information (Fig. 3.2).

Signal-to-noise ratio

The signal-to-noise ratio is the ratio between the wanted information (for example, the image of a bone) and unwanted interference 'noise' (anything that hinders us from seeing the bone clearly).

It is influenced by the following.

- Scatter: in the horse, the major factor causing 'noise' in an image is scatter radiation, which is in turn influenced by the amount and radiodensity of the tissues. This is especially a problem in the proximal area of the horse.
- Collimation: the easiest way to decrease scatter is to collimate as tightly as possible around the area of interest.
- Exposure values: discussed below.
- Detector and post-processing system: some systems are more sensitive to scatter than others.
- Filter: this can be in the form of mechanical grids or digital filters. Grids can be used to reduce scatter to a certain degree. DR systems often reach the same scatter reduction as a grid through inbuilt filters. Grids need to be carefully chosen for the system used and require perfect alignment of the beam and an exact distance between the grid and the X-ray machine (required distance is usually shown on a label on the grid).

Exposures

There are three parameters that determine radiation exposure: kVp (peak kilovoltage), mA (milliamperes) and time (seconds).

- kVp determines the energy of the X-ray beam and its penetration 'power'. Decreasing the kVp settings increases the image contrast and decreases the latitude. A kVp setting under 70 is desirable for good bone radiographs. The higher the kVp, the lower the contrast and the more scatter is generated.
- mAs is the product of time and mA and determines the number of electrons and hence photons. It influences the 'blackness' of radiographs, but not the contrast. As a rule of thumb, it is a good idea to keep the time to under 0.2 seconds to avoid motion artefacts.
- Exposure latitude is the extent to which a radiograph can be over- or underexposed and

still achieve an acceptable result. CR and DR systems have a wide latitude, meaning that over- and underexposures can still result in a diagnostic image thanks to post-processing. Of course, following the ALARA principle one should always aim for the lowest exposure necessary for radiation safety reasons.

- Overexposure on CR and DR systems does not result in a black image like on conventional film–screen systems and to assess exposure one needs to be attentive to certain numeric values (e.g. in the Fuji CR system they are labelled S and L value and they must be within a certain range). These values are recommended by the manufacturer.
- Overexposure can result in an artificial blackness of borders of bones ('blackout'). This may obscure lesions at bone margins and care should be taken that the soft tissue envelope is visible on radiographs to ensure that the true margins of the bones are visible (Fig. 3.3).
- Underexposure often results in a very noisy image, which influences our ability to see trabecular detail and may also obscure lesions; in these cases, an increase in mAs is indicated (Fig. 3.4).
- Portable X-ray machines are low-output generators. The maximum output they are capable of should be displayed on the machine (usually on a little sticker somewhere). Many of these machines will only generate the maximum output for a few times in a short time period before they either stop working for a while or image quality will deteriorate because the machine generates lower outputs.

Image distortion and centring

- Image distortion is influenced by the angle of the X-ray beam to the object and the angle of the X-ray beam to the plate. Ideally, the X-ray beam should be aligned at 90 degrees to the area of interest and the plate to avoid image distortion.

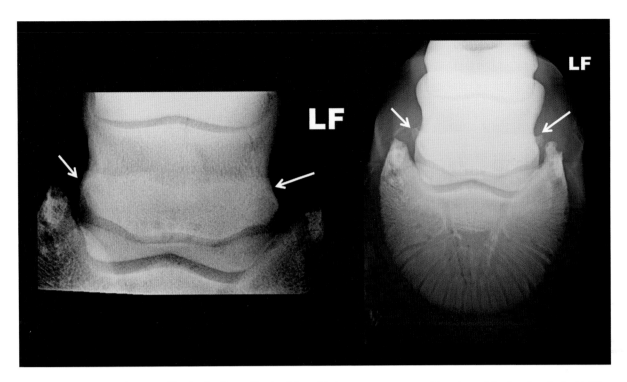

Figure 3.3 These images illustrate the effect of too high exposures resulting in a 'blackout artefact'. The image on the left is a dorsoproximal-palmarodistal radiograph of the navicular bone, where too high exposures have led to a 'blackout' artefact obscuring the lateral and medial edges of the navicular bone. The radiograph on the right is a radiograph of the same foot with lower exposures that shows considerable enthesophyte formation at the attachment of the sesamoidean collateral ligaments (white arrows).

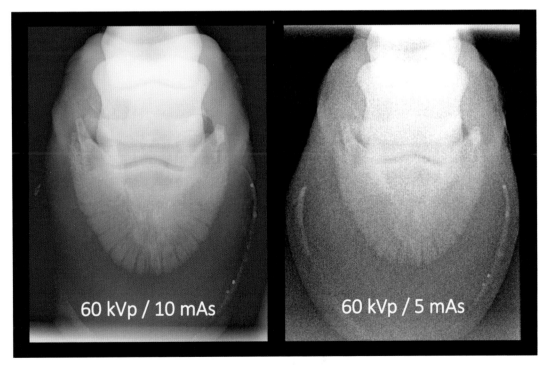

Figure 3.4 This figure illustrates the effect of exposure on the signal-to-noise ratio in an image. These are two dorsoproximal-palmarodistal radiographs of a foot; the image on the left was acquired with 60 kVp and 10 mAs whereas the image on the right was acquired with half the mAs. The image on the right shows more noise that can be appreciated as a speckled pattern and obscures anatomical detail compared to the image on the left where there is less noise and more detail.

- In most applications, we are trying to highlight small details that require the X-ray beam to be orientated tangential to the lesion, e.g. highlighting osteophytes at articular margins or subchondral bone changes. To avoid missing small lesions we use four projections as standard in the horse's leg; in the case of the foot even more. This inevitably means the X-ray beam hits the bone at a degree other than 90 degrees resulting in distortion.
- While we often manage to keep the X-ray beam at 90 degrees to the X-ray plate, this can be compromised, e.g. in a lateromedial stifle this can sometimes not be achieved or in the case where we acquire an upright pedal bone view with the leg standing on a tunnel block.
- Image distortion is also caused by suboptimal centring. In the horse, we usually try to 'shoot' through joint spaces and if we do not manage to align the direction of the beam with the slope of the joint, the joint space will be obscured due to superimposition.
- For many applications we use a horizontal beam in horses, which will work for horizontally orientated joints. Only the central beam is truly horizontal while the other components of an X-ray beam diverge in a cone shape from that. If the beam is not directly centred on the joint, this divergence will result in superimposition of the surrounding structures on the joint space.
- Some joints are naturally sloped (e.g. the distal intertarsal and tarsometatarsal joints slope from lateroproximal to distomedial) and the beam has to be adjusted accordingly.
- It is vital to have the horse standing square and equally weight-bearing to standardize joint alignment as much as possible. Some horses' conformation requires the adjustment of the X-ray beam to their individual leg alignment.

Post-processing artefacts

Post-processing artefacts are often system-specific but include 'overzealous' edge enhancement or noise reduction, which may lead to misinterpretation of trabecular pattern; again, it is a good idea to discuss this with the vendor's applications technician. Different practices have different requirements, e.g. a practice that primarily radiographs racehorses will want to put more emphasis on visualization of changes in bone density and trabecular pattern, which requires 'harder' images with more bone detail and less soft tissue. Whereas a practice that deals with general riding horses may be more interested in visualizing signs of osteoarthritis, such as joint effusion and periarticular osteophytes which require 'softer images' with good detail of joint margins.

Other artefacts

Some of the most annoying artefacts are on the horse and often relatively easy to avoid, for example dirt on the skin or solar surface can mimic lesions. A good wire brush is very helpful to clean the hoof. In heavily feathered horses, feathers and the air between them can obscure lesions. We have found wetting them down smoothly or using a rubber band to keep them away beneficial.

CHAPTER 4

Foot

Indications

Foot diseases are the most common cause of forelimb lameness in the horse, hence radiography of this region is commonly performed in clinical practice.

Indications for performing radiographs of the foot include:

- Lameness localized to the foot by diagnostic analgesia (palmar digital nerve block, basi-sesamoid block, pastern ring block, distal interphalangeal joint block or navicular bursa block)
- Positive response to hoof testers
- Effusion of the distal interphalangeal joint
- Increased digital pulses
- Penetrating injuries to the sole
- Clinical signs of laminitis
- Assessment of foot conformation
- As part of a pre-purchase examination.

Equipment

For a complete study of the foot, specific equipment is required, including:

- Portable X-ray machine
- Farriery kit for shoe removal and hoof preparation
- Play-Doh or similar to pack frog grooves

- Flat blocks to raise feet for the weight-bearing projections
- Tunnel and Hickman blocks
- Plate holder
- Radiation safety equipment: lead gowns, lead gloves and thyroid protectors.

Preparation

Shoes are best removed for foot radiographs, unless:

- The purpose of the radiographs is to assess shoe fit
- The shoes do not interfere with assessment of structures, e.g. conformation assessment
- It is clinically contraindicated to remove shoes, for example in a laminitic horse.

The foot requires cleaning and trimming to reduce artefacts caused by loose horn and dirt.

Packing the frog grooves with a substance of similar opacity to horn (e.g. Play-Doh) will help to eliminate artefacts caused by gas within the grooves (Fig. 4.1). In order to keep the packing in, it is useful to cover the sole with paper or cling film.

Sedation of the patient is advised.

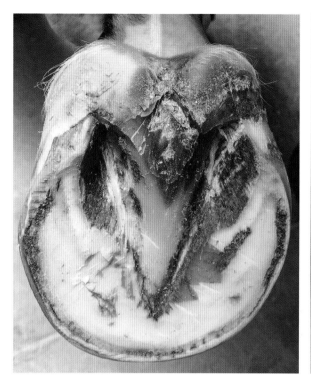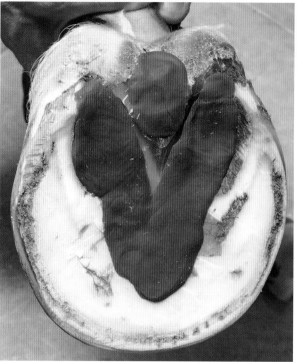

Figure 4.1 Preparation of the foot prior to obtaining radiographs.

Radiographic protocol

A standard radiographic examination of the foot usually includes at least five radiographs, although this may vary depending on the suspected disease:

- Lateromedial (LM)
- Dorsopalmar (DPa)
- Dorsoproximal-palmarodistal oblique (DPr-PaDiO) for the distal phalanx and sole
- Dorsoproximal-palmarodistal oblique (DPr-PaDiO) for the navicular bone
- Palmaroproximal-palmarodistal oblique (PaPr-PaDiO) or 'skyline' view of the navicular bone.

Additional projections:

- Dorso 45° lateral-palmaromedial oblique (D45L-PaMO) and dorso 45° medial-palmarolateral oblique (D45M-PaLO).

Note: when radiographs of the hind foot are obtained, the term palmar should be changed to plantar.

Lateromedial (LM) (Figs 4.2–4.8)

1. Remove shoes unless hoof balance assessment is required.
2. Remove dirt and any loose horn from the sole.
3. Position both feet on flat blocks with each foot at the medial edge of the block.
4. Stand the horse square with the cannon bone vertical to the ground in each direction and ensure all limbs are equally weight-bearing.
5. A marker on the dorsal hoof wall and just in front of the tip of the frog can help in the radiographic assessment of horses with laminitis.
6. Place the plate resting on the ground in landscape orientation on the medial side of the foot, as close as possible to the limb, and lower than the solar surface.
7. Place a R/L marker on the dorsal side of the plate.
8. Position the X-ray machine on the lateral side of the foot.
9. Focus–film distance: 100 cm.
10. The X-ray beam is usually orientated horizontally but depending on a horse's foot conformation, the X-ray beam may have to be angled up or down.
11. Align the beam perpendicular to the limb, parallel to the bulbs of the heel.
12. Centre the X-ray beam at the level of the distal interphalangeal joint, approximately 1 cm below the coronary band, midway between the dorsal hoof wall and the heel.
13. Collimate around the foot, including half of the proximal phalanx.
14. Exposure guide: 65 kVp, 8 mAs.

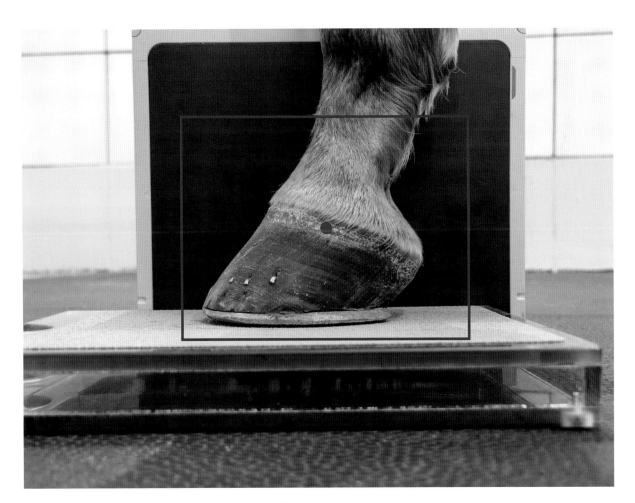

Figure 4.2 Positioning to obtain a LM view of the foot.

Figure 4.3
LM projection of the foot.

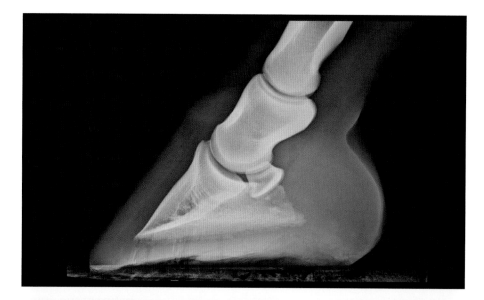

Figure 4.4
Radiographic anatomy of the LM projection of the foot.

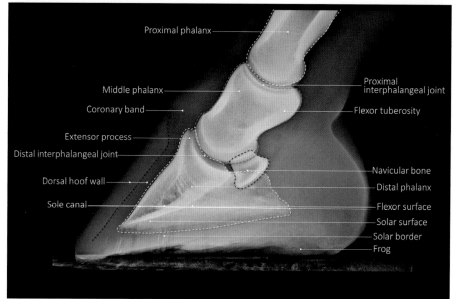

Figure 4.5
3D representation of the LM projection of the foot.

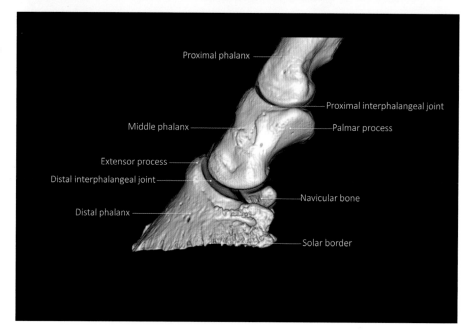

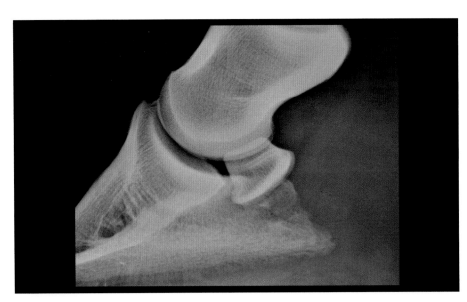

Figure 4.6
LM projection of the navicular bone.

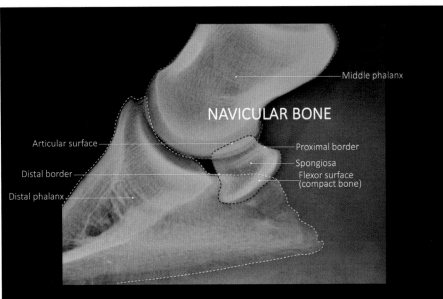

Figure 4.7
Radiographic anatomy of the LM projection of the navicular bone.

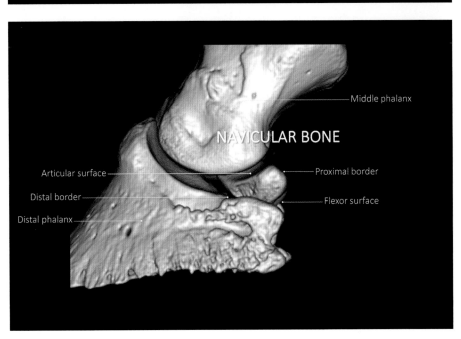

Figure 4.8
3D representation of the LM projection of the navicular bone.

Dorsopalmar (DPa) (Figs 4.9–4.12)

1. Remove shoes unless hoof balance assessment is required.
2. Remove dirt and any loose horn from the sole.
3. Position both feet on flat blocks with the heels at the caudal edge of the block.
4. Stand the horse square with the cannon bone vertical to the ground in each direction, and ensure all limbs are equally weight-bearing.
5. Place the plate resting on the ground in portrait orientation on the palmar side of the foot, as close as possible to the limb, and lower than the solar surface.
6. Place a R/L marker on the lateral side of the plate.
7. Position the X-ray machine on the dorsal side of the foot.
8. Focus–film distance: 100 cm.
9. Use a horizontal X-ray beam.
10. Centre the X-ray beam at the level of the distal interphalangeal joint, approximately 1 cm below the coronary band, in the midline of the hoof.
11. Collimate around the foot, including half of the proximal phalanx.
12. Exposure guide: 65 kVp, 8 mAs.

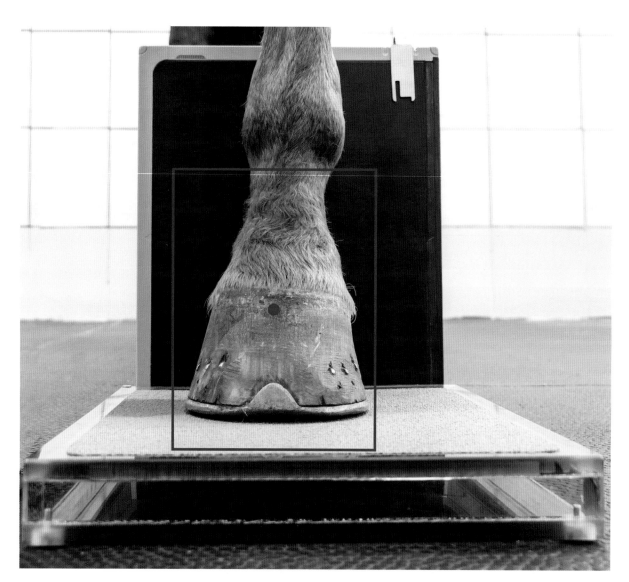

Figure 4.9 Positioning to obtain a DPa view of the foot.

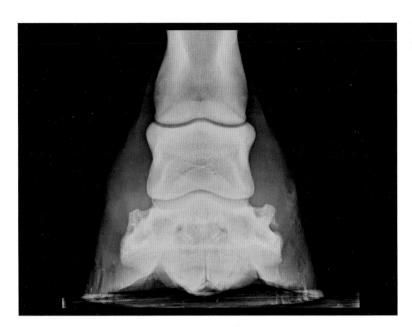

Figure 4.10 DPa projection of the foot.

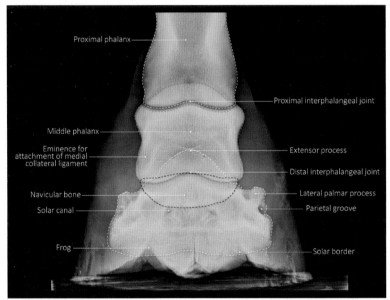

Figure 4.11 Radiographic anatomy of the DPa projection of the foot.

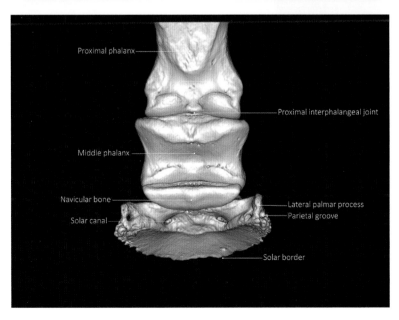

Figure 4.12 3D representation of the DPa projection of the foot.

Dorsoproximal-palmarodistal oblique (DPr-PaDiO) (Figs 4.13–4.20)

This projection is performed twice, once to image the navicular bone and once to image the distal phalanx. Different centring and exposures are used in each projection.

Two different methods can be used to obtain DPr-PaDiO projections:

- High coronary technique: the horse's foot stands on a tunnel block and the X-ray beam is angled downward 65 degrees from the horizontal (Fig. 4.10).
- Upright pedal technique: the horse's foot is positioned with the toe pointing downwards on a Hickman/Oxspring block and a horizontal X-ray beam is used (Fig. 4.11).

High coronary technique

1. Remove shoes.
2. Remove dirt and any loose horn from the sole.
3. Pack the foot with Play-Doh.
4. Stand the horse square with the cannon bone vertical to the ground in each direction, and ensure all limbs are equally weight-bearing.
5. Position the foot being imaged on a tunnel block.
6. Position the contralateral foot on a flat block.
7. Place the plate facing upwards in the tunnel block.
8. Place a R/L marker on the lateral side of the plate.
9. Position the X-ray machine dorsoproximally to the foot.
10. Focus–film distance: 100 cm.
11. Angle the X-ray beam 65 degrees downward from the horizontal.
12. Centre the X-ray beam in the midline of the hoof at:
    - The coronary band for the distal phalanx
    - 1 cm above the coronary band for the navicular bone.
13. Collimation:
    - Around the foot for the distal phalanx
    - Around the navicular bone for the navicular bone.
14. Exposure guide:
    - Distal phalanx: 65 kVp, 8 mAs
    - Navicular bone: 70 kVp, 10 mAs.

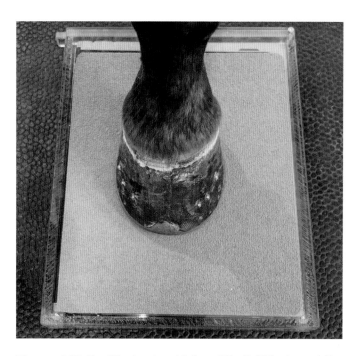

Figure 4.13 Positioning to obtain a DPr-PaDiO view of the foot using a high coronary technique.

Upright pedal technique

1. Remove shoes.
2. Remove dirt and any loose horn from the sole.
3. Pack the foot with Play-Doh.
4. Place the foot with gloved hands on a Hickman block that is positioned slightly forward relative to the horse. The fetlock must be kept as much extended as possible.
5. Place the plate in portrait orientation on the palmar side of the foot as close as possible to the foot.
6. Place a R/L marker on the lateral side of the plate.
7. Position the X-ray machine on the dorsal side of the foot.
8. Focus–film distance: 100 cm.
9. Use a horizontal X-ray beam.
10. Centre the X-ray beam in the midline of the hoof at:
    – The coronary band for the distal phalanx
    – 1 cm above the coronary band for the navicular bone.
11. Collimation:
    – Around the foot for the distal phalanx
    – Around the navicular bone for the navicular bone.
12. Exposure guide:
    – Distal phalanx: 65 kVp, 8 mAs
    – Navicular bone: 70 kVp, 10 mAs.

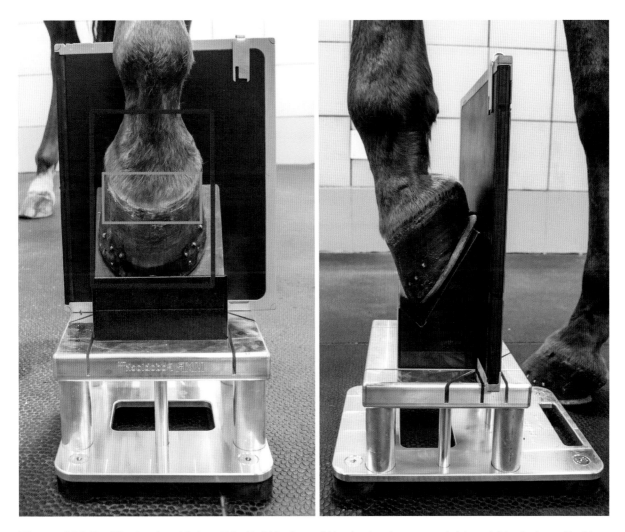

Figure 4.14 Positioning to obtain a DPr-PaDiO view of the foot using an upright pedal technique. Red box represents collimation for the distal phalanx and blue box represents collimation for the navicular bone.

Figure 4.15 DPr-PaDiO projection of the distal phalanx.

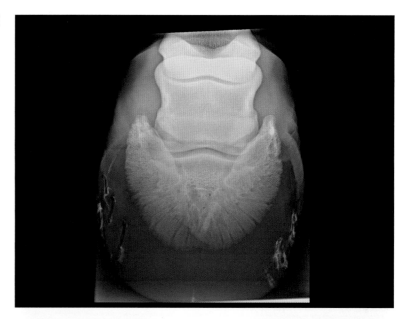

Figure 4.16 Radiographic anatomy of the DPr-PaDiO projection of the distal phalanx.

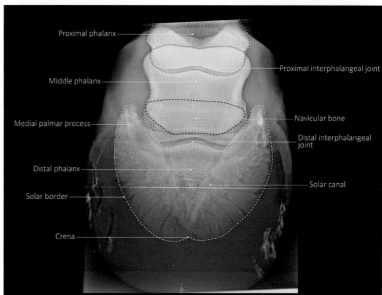

Figure 4.17 3D representation of the DPr-PaDiO projection of the distal phalanx.

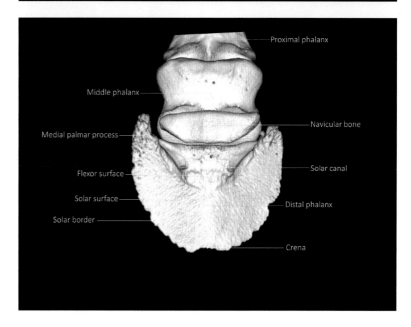

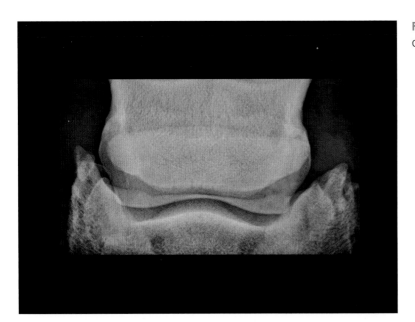

Figure 4.18 DPr-PaDiO projection of the navicular bone.

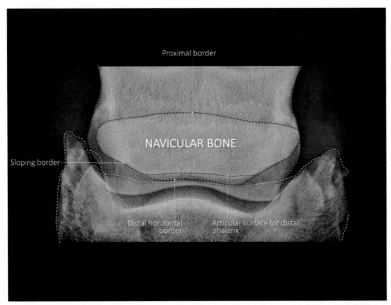

Figure 4.19 Radiographic anatomy of the DPr-PaDiO projection of the navicular bone.

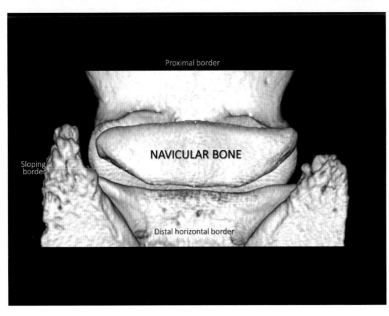

Figure 4.20 3D representation of the DPr-PaDiO projection of the navicular bone.

Palmaroproximal-palmarodistal oblique (PaPr-PaDiO) or 'skyline' view of the navicular bone (Figs 4.21–4.24)

1. Remove shoes.
2. Remove dirt and any loose horn from the sole.
3. Pack the foot with Play-Doh.
4. Position the foot being imaged on a tunnel block as far back underneath the horse as possible while still keeping the foot weight-bearing. It is also helpful in some horses to position the foot slightly turned outward.
5. Place the plate facing upwards in the tunnel block.
6. Place a R/L marker on the lateral side of the plate.
7. Position the X-ray machine under the abdomen of the horse. A 100 cm focus–film distance is usually not possible since the X-ray machine cannot be positioned high enough.
8. Angle the X-ray beam downward hitting the foot at 45 degrees from the horizontal. A low-heel foot conformation may require a slightly more horizontal X-ray beam angle.
9. Centre the X-ray beam just proximal to the bulbs of the heel, without superimposing the palmar aspect of the fetlock on the image.
10. Collimate tightly around the navicular bone to reduce scatter.
11. Exposure guide: 75 kVp, 8 mAs.

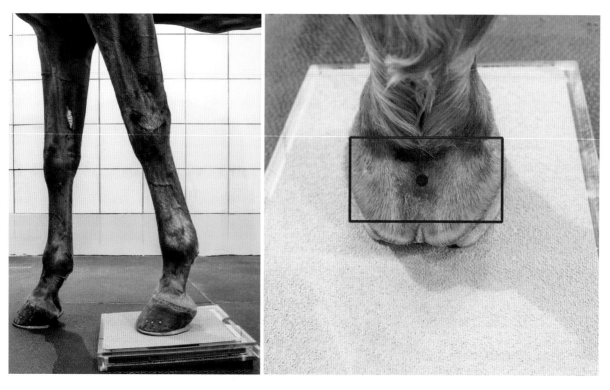

Figure 4.21 Positioning to obtain a PaPr-PaDiO view of the foot.

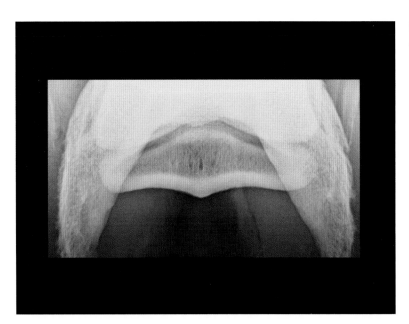

Figure 4.22 PaPr-PaDiO projection of the foot.

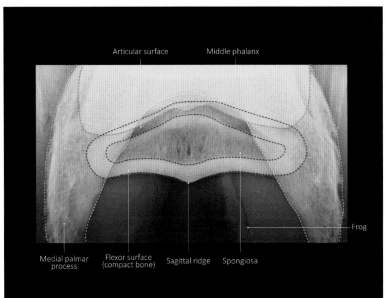

Figure 4.23 Radiographic anatomy of the PaPr-PaDiO projection of the foot.

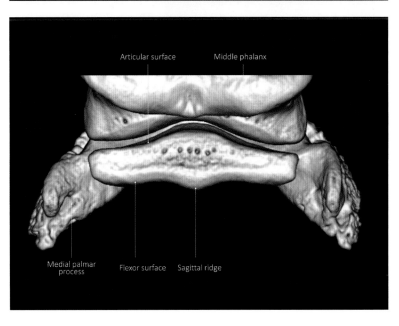

Figure 4.24 3D representation of the PaPr-PaDiO projection of the foot.

Dorso 45° lateral-palmaromedial oblique (D45L-PaMO) and dorso 45° medial-palmarolateral oblique (D45M-PaLO) (Figs 4.25–4.28)

1. Remove shoes.
2. Remove dirt and any loose horn from the sole.
3. Pack the foot with Play-Doh.
4. Place the foot with gloved hands on a Hickman block that is positioned slightly forward relative to the horse. The fetlock must be kept as much extended as possible.
5. Place the plate in portrait orientation with a R/L marker on its lateral side.

   – D45L-PaMO: highlights the lateral palmar process of the distal phalanx. The X-ray machine is positioned on the dorsolateral side of the foot, at a 45-degree angle from the sagittal plane of the limb. The plate is perpendicular to the X-ray beam on the palmaromedial side of the leg.
   – D45M-PaLO: highlights the medial palmar process of the distal phalanx. The X-ray machine is positioned on the dorsomedial side of the foot, at a 45-degree angle from the sagittal plane of the limb. The plate is perpendicular to the X-ray beam on the palmarolateral side of the leg.

Alternatively, a 60-degree angle from the sagittal plane of the limb can be used when evaluation of the articular margins and extensor process of the distal phalanx is required.

6. Focus–film distance: 100 cm.
7. Use a horizontal X-ray beam.
8. Centre the X-ray beam at the coronary band on the lateral or the medial hoof wall for the D45L-PaMO or the D45M-PaLO, respectively.
9. Collimate around the foot.
10. Exposure guide: 70 kVp, 8 mAs.

Note: Alternatively, a Pr45L-DiMO and a Pr45M-DiLO can be obtained to image the lateral and medial palmar processes, respectively. The horse stands on a tunnel block, the X-ray machine is placed on the lateral or lateral side of the limb and the X-ray beam is angled 45 degrees downward from the horizontal.

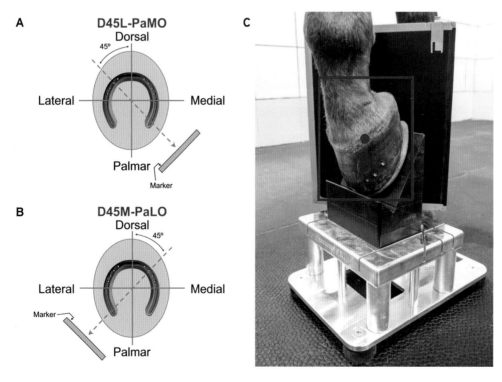

Figure 4.25 Diagram showing how to obtain D45L-PaMO (A) and D45M-PaLO (B) views of the foot and positioning to obtain a D45L-PaMO view of the foot (C).

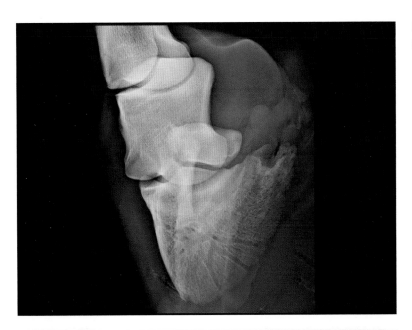

Figure 4.26 D45L-PaMO projection of the foot.

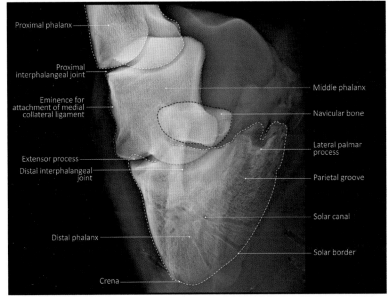

Figure 4.27 Radiographic anatomy of the D45L-PaMO projection of the foot.

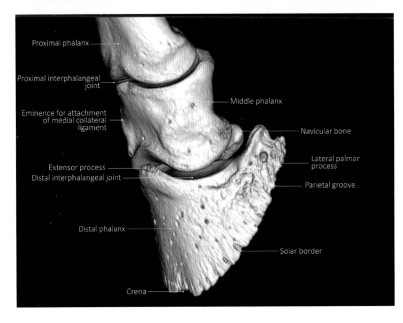

Figure 4.28 3D representation of the D45L-PaMO projection of the foot.

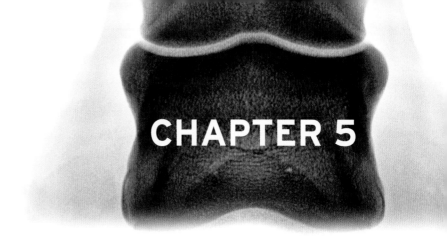

CHAPTER 5

Pastern

Indications

Indications for performing radiographs of the pastern include:

- Lameness localized to the pastern by diagnostic analgesia (abaxial nerve block, basisesamoid block, pastern ring block or proximal inter-phalangeal joint block)
- Positive flexion test
- Soft tissue and bony swellings
- Effusion of the pastern joint
- Effusion of the digital flexor tendon sheath
- Pastern lacerations
- As part of a pre-purchase examination.

Equipment

For a complete study of the pastern the following equipment is required:

- Portable X-ray machine
- Flat blocks to raise feet
- Plate holder
- Radiation safety equipment: lead gowns, lead gloves and thyroid protectors.

Preparation

If necessary, brush or wash the area to reduce artefacts caused by dirt. Sedation of the patient is advised. In heavily feathered horses it can be helpful to wet down the coat, plait the hair or bandage it.

Radiographic protocol

A standard radiographic examination of the pastern usually includes four projections:

- Lateromedial (LM)
- Dorsopalmar (DPa)
- Dorso 45° lateral-palmaromedial oblique (D45L-PaMO) and dorso 45° medial-palmarolateral oblique (D45M-PaLO).

Note: when radiographs of the hind pastern are obtained, the term palmar should be changed to plantar.

Lateromedial (LM) (Figs 5.1–5.4)

1. Stand the horse square with the cannon bone vertical to the ground in each direction, and ensure all limbs are equally weight-bearing.
2. Position both feet on flat blocks with each foot at the medial edge of the block.
3. Place the plate resting on the ground in portrait orientation on the medial side of the limb, as close as possible to the foot.
4. Place a R/L marker on the dorsal aspect of the plate.
5. Position the X-ray machine on the lateral side of the limb.
6. Focus–film distance: 100 cm.
7. Use a horizontal X-ray beam.
8. Align the beam perpendicular to the limb, parallel to bulbs of the heel.
9. Centre the X-ray beam at the level of the proximal interphalangeal joint, midway between the coronary band and the fetlock.
10. Collimate around the pastern region.
11. Exposure guide: 65 kVp, 8 mAs.

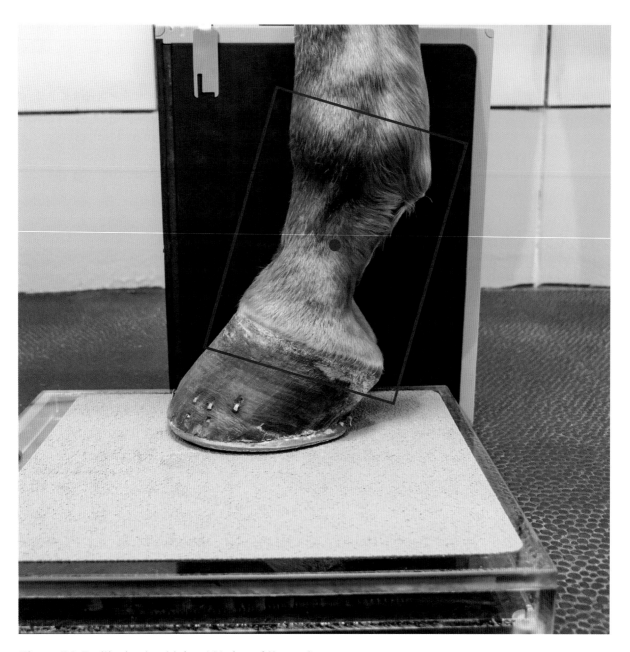

Figure 5.1 Positioning to obtain a LM view of the pastern.

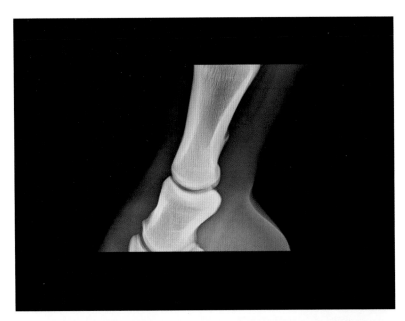

Figure 5.2 LM projection of the pastern.

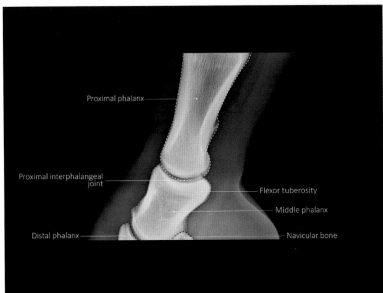

Figure 5.3 Radiographic anatomy of the LM projection of the pastern.

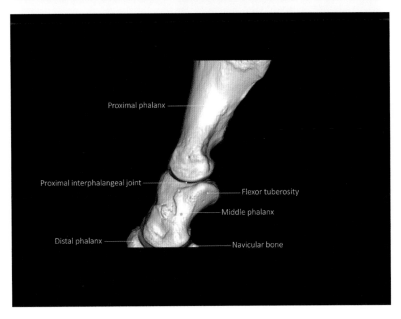

Figure 5.4 3D representation of the LM projection of the pastern.

Dorsopalmar (DPa) (Figs 5.5–5.8)

1. Stand the horse square with the cannon bone vertical to the ground in each direction, and ensure all limbs are equally weight-bearing.
2. Position both feet on flat blocks with the heels at the caudal edge of the block.
3. Place the plate resting on the ground in portrait orientation on the palmar side of the limb, as close as possible to the foot. The plate should be angled parallel to the pastern axis.
4. Place a R/L marker on the lateral side of the plate.
5. Position the X-ray machine on the dorsal side of the foot.
6. Focus–film distance: 100 cm.
7. Angle the X-ray beam 5–10 degrees downward from the horizontal.
8. Centre the X-ray beam at the level of the proximal interphalangeal joint, midway between the coronary band and the fetlock.
9. Collimate around the pastern region.
10. Exposure guide: 65 kVp, 8 mAs.

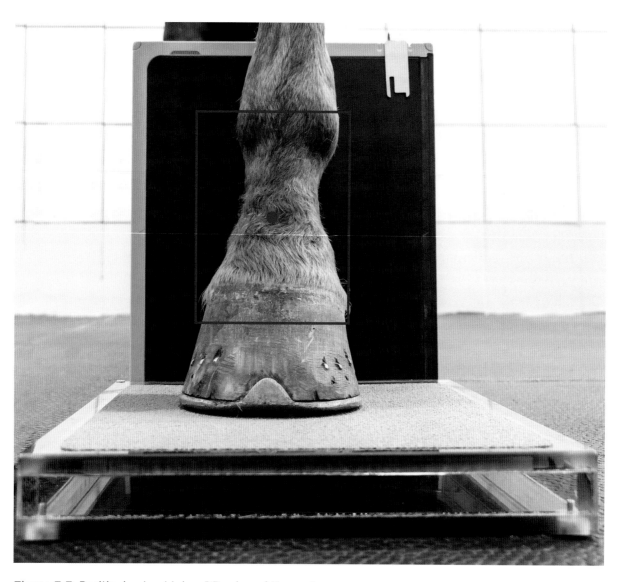

Figure 5.5 Positioning to obtain a DPa view of the pastern.

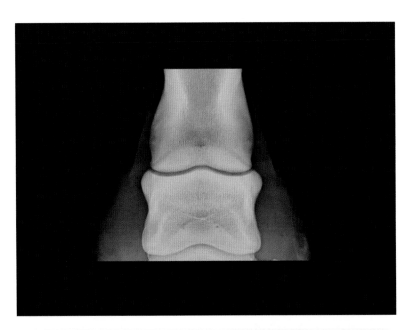

Figure 5.6 DPa projection of the pastern.

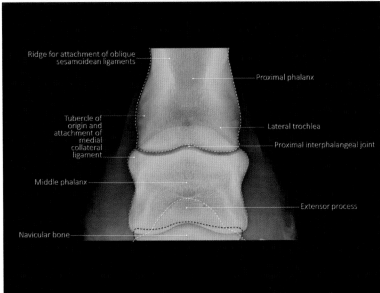

Figure 5.7 Radiographic anatomy of the DPa projection of the pastern.

Ridge for attachment of oblique sesamoidean ligaments

Proximal phalanx

Tubercle of origin and attachment of medial collateral ligament

Lateral trochlea

Proximal interphalangeal joint

Middle phalanx

Extensor process

Navicular bone

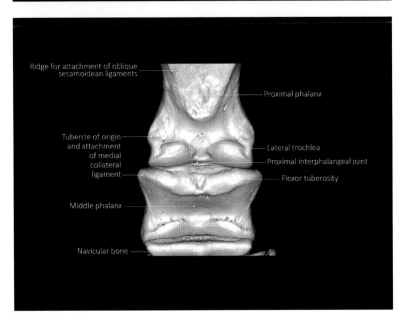

Figure 5.8 3D representation of the DPa projection of the pastern.

Ridge for attachment of oblique sesamoidean ligaments

Proximal phalanx

Tubercle of origin and attachment of medial collateral ligament

Lateral trochlea

Proximal interphalangeal joint

Flexor tuberosity

Middle phalanx

Navicular bone

Dorso 45° lateral-palmaromedial oblique (D45L-PaMO) and dorso 45° medial-palmarolateral oblique (D45M-PaLO) (Figs 5.9–5.12)

1. Stand the horse square with the cannon bone vertical to the ground in each direction, and ensure all limbs are equally weight-bearing.
2. Position both feet on flat blocks with the heels at the caudal edge of the block.
3. Place the plate resting on the ground in portrait orientation with a R/L marker on its lateral side.

   – D45L-PaMO: the X-ray machine is positioned on the dorsolateral side of the joint, at a 45-degree angle from the sagittal plane of the limb. The plate is perpendicular to the X-ray beam on the palmaromedial side of the leg.
   – D45M-PaLO: the X-ray machine is positioned on the dorsomedial side of the joint, at a 45-degree angle from the sagittal plane of the limb. The plate is perpendicular to the X-ray beam on the palmarolateral side of the leg.

4. Focus–film distance: 100 cm.
5. Use a horizontal X-ray beam.
6. Centre the X-ray beam at the level of the proximal interphalangeal joint, midway between the coronary band and the fetlock.
7. Collimate around the pastern region.
8. Exposure guide: 65 kVp, 8 mAs.

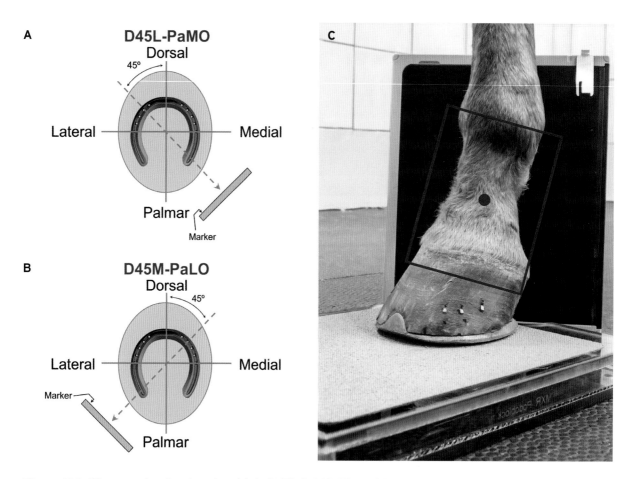

Figure 5.9 Diagram showing how to obtain D45L-PaMO (A) and D45M-PaLO (B) views of the pastern and positioning to obtain a D45L-PaMO view of the pastern (C).

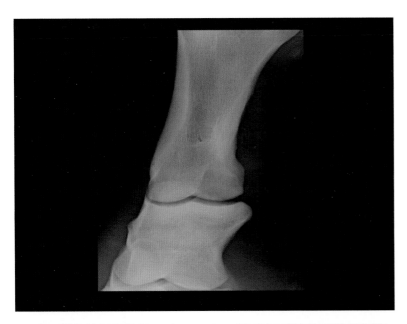

Figure 5.10 D45L-PaMO projection of the pastern.

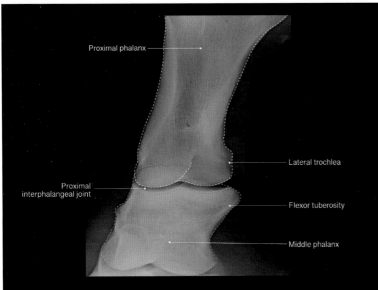

Figure 5.11 Radiographic anatomy of the D45L-PaMO projection of the pastern.

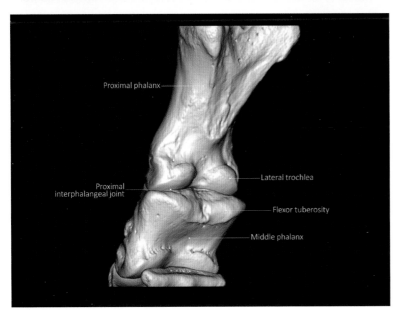

Figure 5.12 3D representation of the D45L-PaMO projection of the pastern.

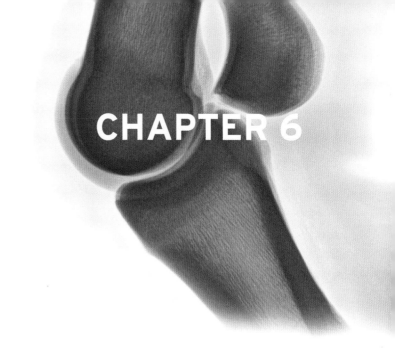

Fetlock

CHAPTER 6

Indications

Fetlock diseases are a common cause of lameness in the horse and therefore radiography of this region is a routine procedure performed in equine practice.

Indications for performing radiographs of the fetlock include:

- Lameness localized to the fetlock by diagnostic analgesia (low four-point nerve block or fetlock joint block)
- Positive flexion test
- Soft tissue swellings, including effusion of the fetlock joint and digital flexor tendon sheath
- Signs of trauma, including wounds and swellings
- As part of a pre-purchase or pre-sales examination.

Equipment

For a complete study of the fetlock the following equipment is required:

- Portable X-ray machine
- Tunnel and Hickman blocks
- Plate holder
- Radiation safety equipment: lead gowns, lead gloves and thyroid protectors.

Preparation

If necessary, brush or wash the area to reduce artefacts caused by dirt. Sedation of the patient is advised. In heavily feathered horses it is advisable to wet the area down, braid the feathers or bandage it (bearing in mind that this may cause artefacts).

Radiographic protocol

A standard radiographic examination of the fetlock includes four projections:

- Lateromedial (LM)
- Dorsopalmar (DPa)
- Dorso 45° lateral-palmaromedial oblique (D45L-PaMO) and dorso 45° medial-palmarolateral oblique (D45M-PaLO).

Additional projections:

- Flexed lateromedial (flexed LM)
- Dorsoproximal-dorsodistal oblique (DPr-DDiO)
- Palmaroproximal-palmarodistal oblique (PaPr-PaDiO)
- Proximo 45° lateral-distomedial oblique (Pr45L-DiMO) and proximo 45° medial-distolateral oblique (Pr45M-DiLO)
- Dorso 45° proximo 45° lateral-palmaro-

distomedial oblique (D45Pr45L-PaDiMO) and dorso 45° proximo 45° medial-palmarodistolateral oblique (D45Pr45M-PaDiLO)

- Dorso 30° proximo 70° lateral-palmarodistomedial oblique (D30Pr70L- PaDiMO) and dorso 30° proximo 70° medial-palmarodistolateral oblique (D30Pr70M-PaDiLO)

- Flexed dorsopalmar (flexed DPa)
- Dorsodistal-palmaroproximal oblique (DDi-PaPrO).

Note: when the radiographs of the hind fetlock are obtained, the term palmar should be changed to plantar.

Lateromedial (LM) (Figs 6.1–6.4)

1. Stand the horse square with the cannon bone vertical to the ground in each direction, and ensure all limbs are equally weight-bearing.
2. Place the plate resting on the ground in portrait orientation on the medial side of the joint, as close as possible to the limb.
3. Place a R/L marker on the dorsal side of the plate.
4. Position the X-ray machine on the lateral side of the limb.
5. Focus–film distance: 100 cm.
6. Use a horizontal X-ray beam.
7. Align the beam perpendicular to the limb.
8. Centre the X-ray beam at the level of the fetlock joint.
9. Collimate around the fetlock joint.
10. Exposure guide: 65 kVp, 8 mAs.

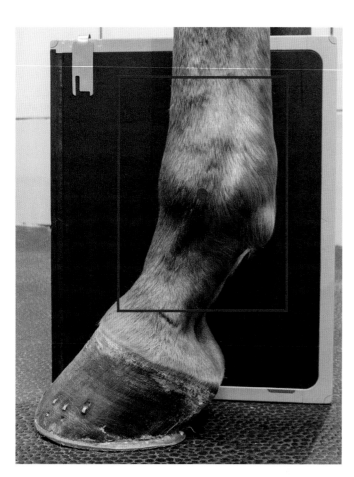

Figure 6.1 Positioning to obtain a LM view of the fetlock.

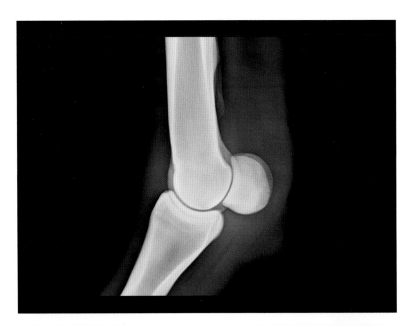

Figure 6.2 LM projection of the fetlock.

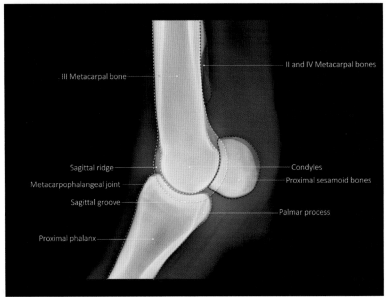

Figure 6.3 Radiographic anatomy of the LM projection of the fetlock.

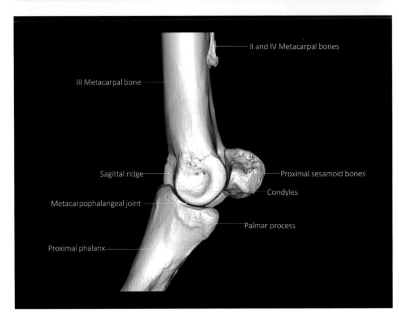

Figure 6.4 3D representation of the LM projection of the fetlock.

Dorsopalmar (DPa) (Figs 6.5–6.8)

1. Stand the horse square with the cannon bone vertical to the ground in each direction, and ensure all limbs are equally weight-bearing.
2. Place the plate resting on the ground in portrait orientation on the palmar side of the joint, as close as possible to the limb. The plate should be aligned parallel with the pastern axis.
3. Place a R/L marker on the lateral side of the plate.
4. Position the X-ray machine on the dorsal side of the limb.
5. Focus–film distance: 100 cm.
6. Angle the X-ray beam 10–15 degrees downward from the horizontal to move the proximal sesamoid bones away from the joint.
7. Centre the X-ray beam at the level of the fetlock joint.
8. Collimate around the fetlock joint.
9. Exposure guide: 70 kVp, 8 mAs.

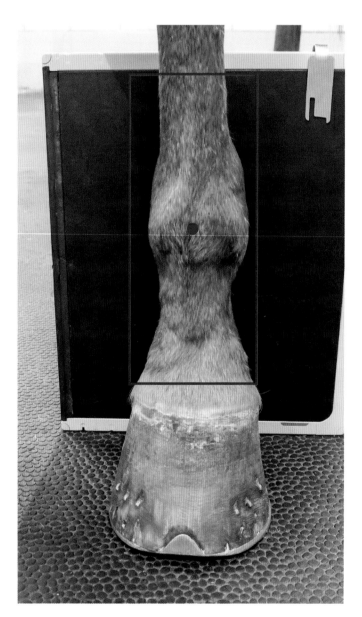

Figure 6.5 Positioning to obtain a DPa view of the fetlock.

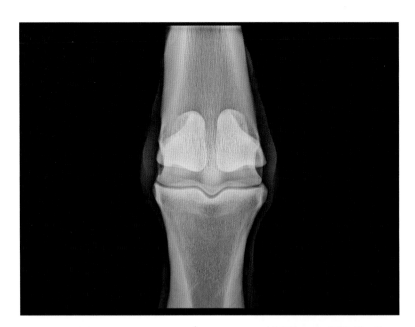

Figure 6.6 DPa projection of the fetlock.

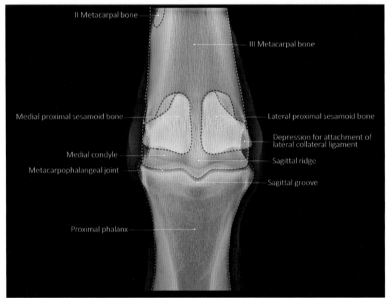

Figure 6.7 Radiographic anatomy of the DPa projection of the fetlock.

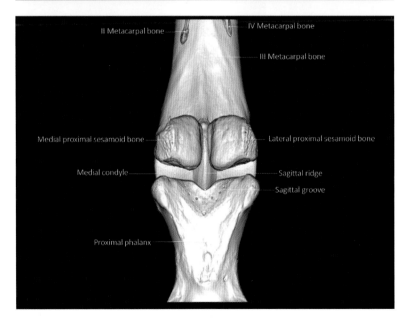

Figure 6.8 3D representation of the DPa projection of the fetlock.

Dorso 45° lateral-palmaromedial oblique (D45L-PaMO) and dorso 45° medial-palmarolateral oblique (D45M-PaLO) (Figs 6.9–6.12)

1. Stand the horse square with the cannon bone vertical to the ground in each direction, and ensure all limbs are equally weight-bearing.
2. Place the plate resting on the ground in portrait orientation with a R/L marker on its lateral side.

   – D45L-PaMO: highlights the lateral proximal sesamoid bone. The X-ray machine is positioned on the dorsolateral side of the joint, at a 45-degree angle from the sagittal plane of the limb. The plate is perpendicular to the X-ray beam on the palmaromedial side of the leg.

   – D45M-PaLO: highlights the medial proximal sesamoid bone. The X-ray machine is positioned on the dorsomedial side of the joint, at a 45-degree angle from the sagittal plane of the limb. The plate is perpendicular to the X-ray beam on the palmarolateral side of the leg.

3. Focus–film distance: 100 cm.
4. Use a horizontal X-ray beam, although this projection can also be obtained by angling the X-ray beam down approximately 10–15 degrees from the horizontal.
5. Centre the X-ray beam at the level of the fetlock joint.
6. Collimate around the fetlock joint.
7. Exposure guide: 65 kVp, 8 mAs.

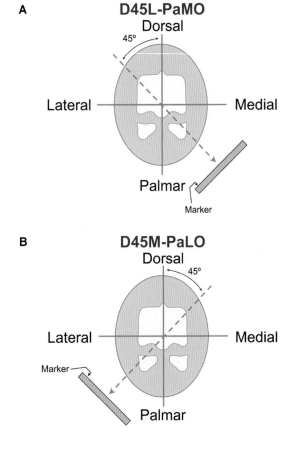

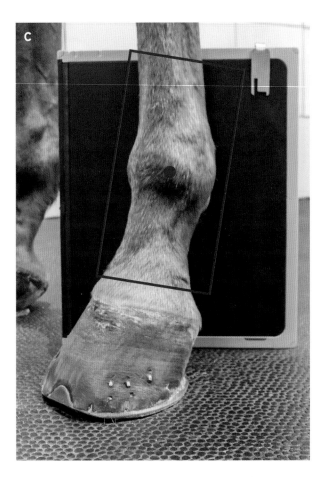

Figure 6.9 Diagram showing how to obtain D45L-PaMO (A) and D45M-PaLO (B) views of the fetlock and positioning to obtain a D45L-PaMO view of the fetlock (C).

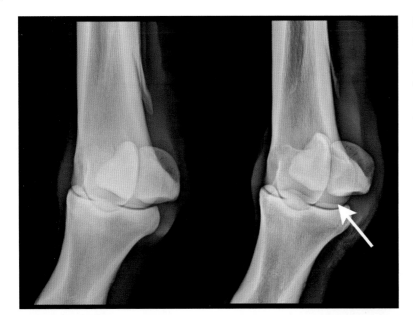

Figure 6.10 D45L-PaMO projections of the fetlock with a horizontal X-ray beam (left) and angling downward 10 degrees from the horizontal (right), which improves assessment of the condyle of the third metacarpal bone (arrow).

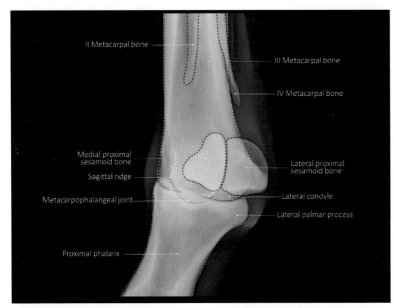

Figure 6.11 Radiographic anatomy of the D45L-PaMO projection of the fetlock.

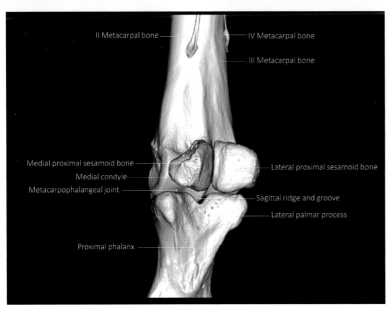

Figure 6.12 3D representation of the D45L-PaMO projection of the fetlock.

Flexed lateromedial (flexed LM) (Figs 6.13–6.16)

1. Flex the fetlock joint and rest the foot onto a Hickman block. Use gloved hands for limb positioning.
2. Place the plate in landscape orientation on the medial side of the joint, as close as possible to the limb.
3. Place a R/L marker on the dorsal side of the plate.
4. Position the X-ray machine on the lateral side of the limb.
5. Focus–film distance: 100 cm.
6. Use a horizontal X-ray beam.
7. Align the beam perpendicular to the limb and the plate.
8. Centre the X-ray beam at the level of the fetlock joint.
9. Collimate around the fetlock joint.
10. Exposure guide: 65 kVp, 8 mAs.

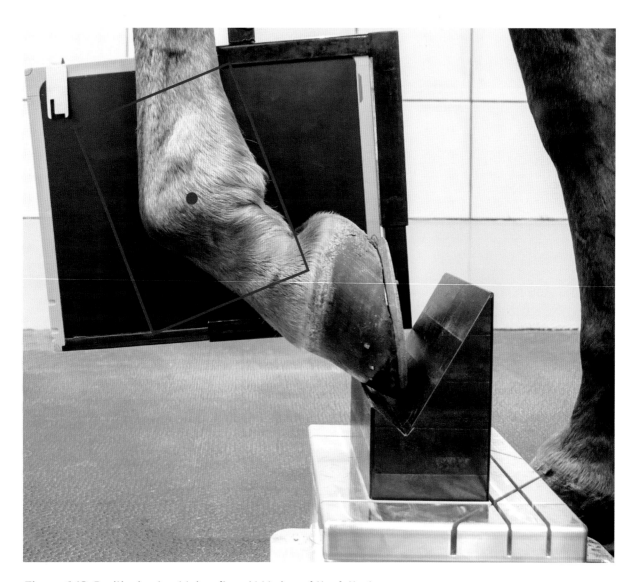

Figure 6.13 Positioning to obtain a flexed LM view of the fetlock.

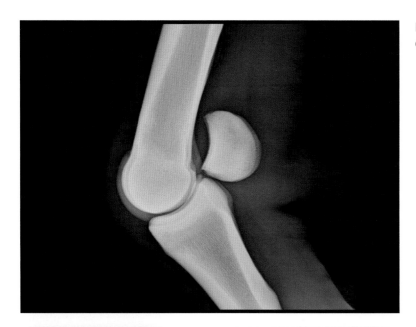

Figure 6.14 Flexed LM projection of the fetlock.

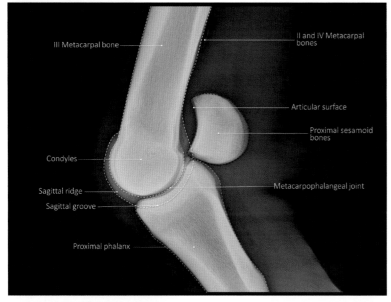

Figure 6.15 Radiographic anatomy of the flexed LM projection of the fetlock.

III Metacarpal bone

II and IV Metacarpal bones

Articular surface

Proximal sesamoid bones

Condyles

Sagittal ridge

Sagittal groove

Metacarpophalangeal joint

Proximal phalanx

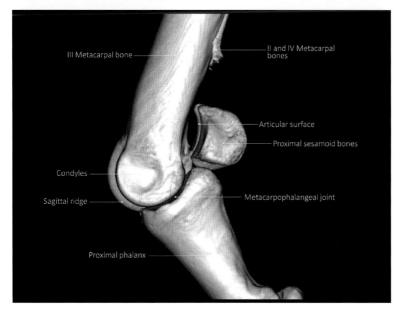

Figure 6.16 3D representation of the flexed LM projection of the fetlock.

III Metacarpal bone

II and IV Metacarpal bones

Articular surface

Proximal sesamoid bones

Condyles

Sagittal ridge

Metacarpophalangeal joint

Proximal phalanx

Dorsoproximal-dorsodistal oblique (DPr-DDiO) (Figs 6.17–6.20)

1. Flex the fetlock joint with gloved hand and keep the metacarpus vertical to the ground.
2. Place the plate distal to the joint, parallel to the ground and facing upwards, as close as possible to the limb.
3. Place a R/L marker on the lateral side of the plate.
4. Position the X-ray machine dorsal to the limb and proximal to the fetlock.
5. Focus–film distance: 100 cm.
6. Angle the X-ray beam 45–70 degrees downward from the horizontal.
7. Centre the X-ray beam at the level of the dorsal aspect of the fetlock joint.
8. Collimate around the fetlock joint.
9. Exposure guide: 60 kVp, 8 mAs.

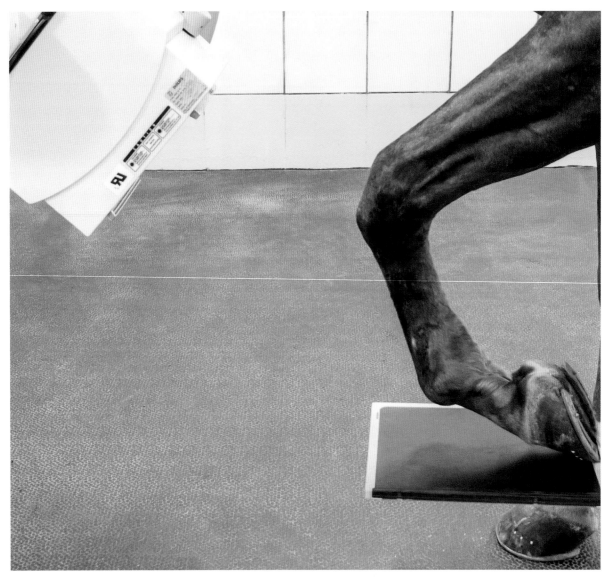

Figure 6.17 Positioning to obtain a DPr-DDiO view of the fetlock.

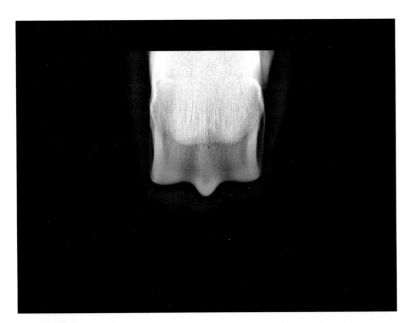

Figure 6.18 DPr-DDiO projection of the fetlock.

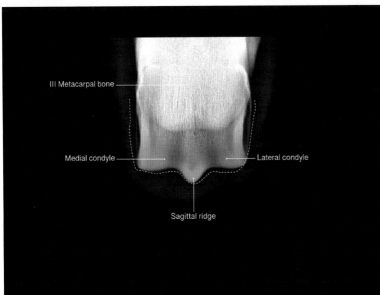

Figure 6.19 Radiographic anatomy of the DPr-DDiO projection of the fetlock.

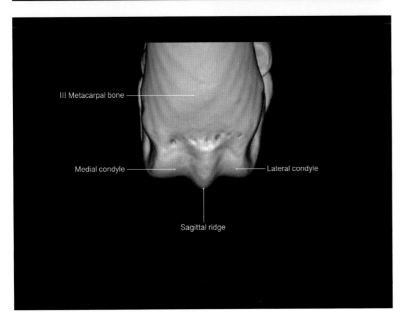

Figure 6.20 3D representation of the DPr-DDiO projection of the fetlock.

Palmaroproximal-palmarodistal oblique (PaPr-PaDiO) (Figs 6.21-6.24)

1. Position the foot being imaged on a tunnel block slightly backward relative to the contralateral limb. The fetlock should be as much extended as possible.
2. Place the plate facing upwards in the tunnel block.
3. Place a R/L marker on the lateral side of the plate.
4. Position the X-ray machine palmar to the limb and proximal to the proximal sesamoid bones. A 100 cm focus–film distance is usually not possible since the X-ray machine cannot be positioned high enough.
5. Angle the X-ray beam 85 degrees downward from the horizontal.
6. Centre the X-ray beam at the level of the proximal sesamoid bones.
7. Collimate around the fetlock joint.
8. Exposure guide: 60 kVp, 8 mAs.

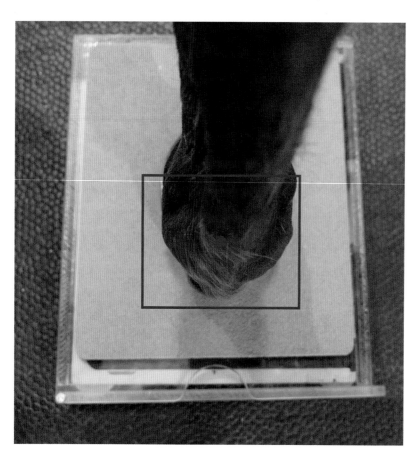

Figure 6.21 Positioning to obtain a PaPr-PaDiO view of the fetlock.

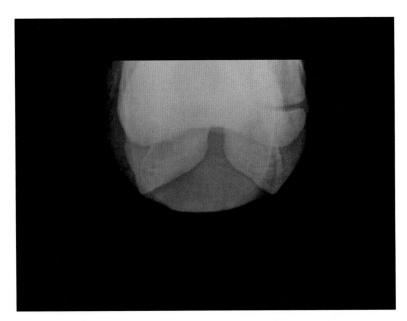

Figure 6.22 PaPr-PaDiO projection of the fetlock.

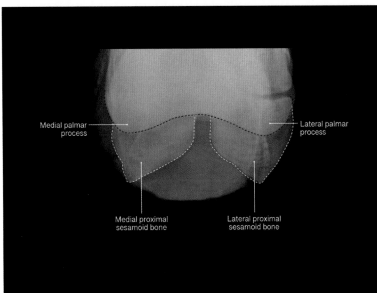

Medial palmar process

Lateral palmar process

Medial proximal sesamoid bone

Lateral proximal sesamoid bone

Figure 6.23 Radiographic anatomy of the PaPr-PaDiO projection of the fetlock.

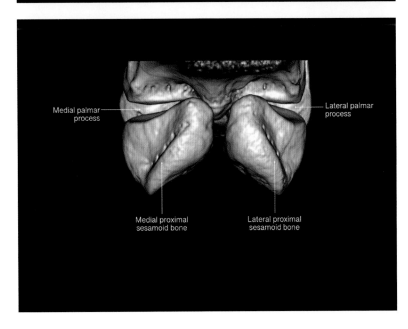

Medial palmar process

Lateral palmar process

Medial proximal sesamoid bone

Lateral proximal sesamoid bone

Figure 6.24 3D representation of the PaPr-PaDiO projection of the fetlock.

Proximo 45° lateral-distomedial oblique (Pr45L-DiMO) and proximo 45° medial-distolateral oblique (Pr45M-DiLO) (Figs 6.25–6.28)

1. Stand the horse square with the cannon bone vertical to the ground in each direction, and ensure all limbs are equally weight-bearing. For the Pr45M-DiLO, the contralateral limb is placed slightly forward or backward to facilitate X-ray tube positioning and avoid superimposition.
2. Place the plate resting on the ground in portrait orientation, as close as possible to the limb.

   – Pr45L-DiMO: the medial proximal sesamoid bone is projected proximally. The X-ray machine is positioned on the lateral side of the joint while the plate is on the medial side.
   – Pr45M-DiLO: the lateral proximal sesamoid bone is projected proximally. The X-ray machine is positioned on the medial side of the joint while the plate is on the lateral side.

3. Focus–film distance: 100 cm.
4. Angle the X-ray beam 45 degrees downward from the horizontal.
5. Centre the X-ray beam at the level of the proximal aspect of the proximal sesamoid bone closer to the tube.
6. Collimate around the fetlock joint.
7. Exposure guide: 65 kVp, 8 mAs.

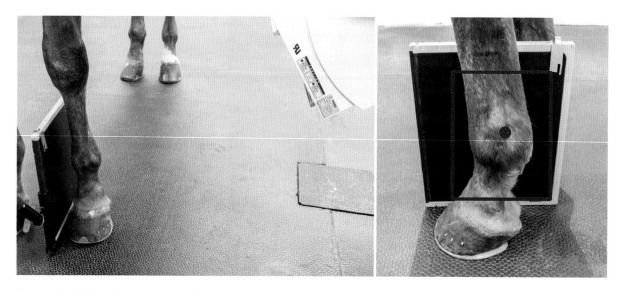

Figure 6.25 Positioning to obtain an Pr45L-DiMO view of the fetlock.

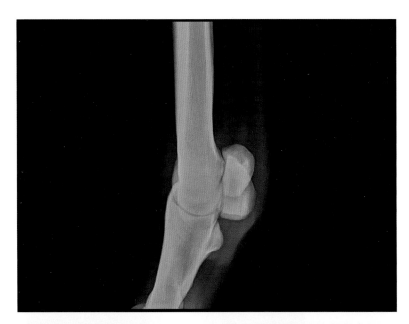

Figure 6.26 Pr45L-DiMO projection of the fetlock.

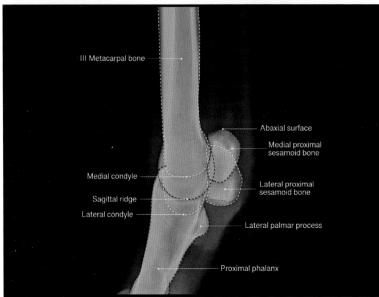

Figure 6.27 Radiographic anatomy of the Pr45L-DiMO projection of the fetlock.

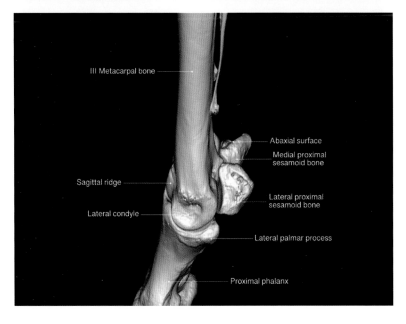

Figure 6.28 3D representation of the Pr45L-DiMO projection of the fetlock.

Dorso 45º proximo 45º lateral-palmarodistomedial oblique (D45Pr45L-PaDiMO) and dorso 45º proximo 45º medial-palmarodistolateral oblique (D45Pr45M-PaDiLO) (Figs 6.29 and 6.30)

1. Stand the horse square with the cannon bone vertical to the ground in each direction, and ensure all limbs are equally weight-bearing.
2. Place the plate resting on the ground in portrait orientation with a R/L marker on its lateral side.

   – D45Pr45L-PaDiMO: highlights the palmar aspect of the lateral condyle of the third metacarpal bone. The X-ray machine is positioned on the dorsolateral side of the joint, at a 45-degree angle from the sagittal plane of the limb. The plate is perpendicular to the X-ray beam on the palmaromedial side of the leg.
   – D45Pr45M-PaDiLO: highlights the palmar aspect of the medial condyle of the third metacarpal bone. The X-ray machine is positioned on the dorsomedial side of the joint, at a 45-degree angle from the sagittal plane of the limb. The plate is perpendicular to the X-ray beam on the palmarolateral side of the leg.

3. Focus–film distance: 100 cm.
4. Angle the X-ray beam 45 degrees downward from the horizontal.
5. Centre the X-ray beam at the level of the fetlock joint.
6. Collimate around the fetlock joint.
7. Exposure guide: 70 kVp, 8 mAs.

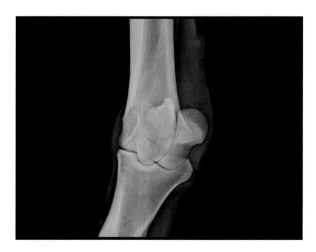

Figure 6.30 D45Pr45L-PaDiMO projection of the fetlock.

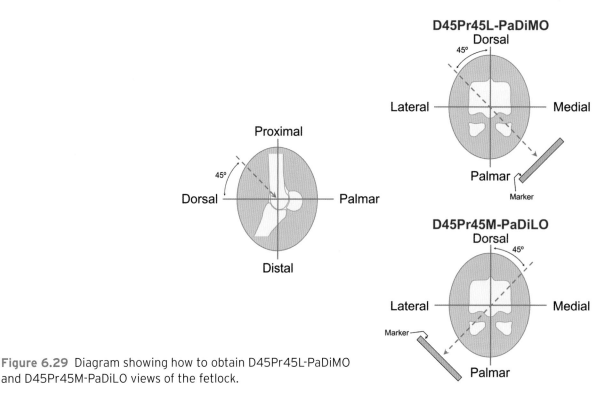

Figure 6.29 Diagram showing how to obtain D45Pr45L-PaDiMO and D45Pr45M-PaDiLO views of the fetlock.

Dorso 30° proximo 70° lateral-palmarodistomedial oblique (D30Pr70L-PaDiMO) and dorso 30° proximo 70° medial-palmarodistolateral oblique (D30Pr70M-PaDiLO) (Figs 6.31 and 6.32)

1. Stand the horse square with the cannon bone vertical to the ground in each direction, and ensure all limbs are equally weight-bearing.
2. Place the plate resting on the ground in portrait orientation with a R/L marker on its lateral side.

   – D30Pr70L-PaDiMO: highlights the lateral palmar process of the proximal phalanx. The X-ray machine is positioned on the dorsolateral side of the joint, at a 70-degree angle from the sagittal plane of the limb. The plate is perpendicular to the X-ray beam on the palmaromedial side of the leg.
   – D30Pr70M-PaDiLO: highlights the medial palmar process of the proximal phalanx. The X-ray machine is positioned on the dorsomedial side of the joint, at a 70-degree angle from the sagittal plane of the limb. The plate is perpendicular to the X-ray beam on the palmarolateral side of the leg.

3. Focus–film distance: 100 cm.
4. Angle the X-ray beam 30 degrees downward from the horizontal.
5. Centre the X-ray beam at the level of the fetlock joint.
6. Collimate around the fetlock joint.
7. Exposure guide: 70 kVp, 8 mAs.

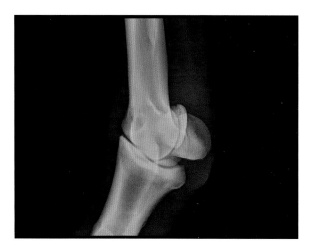

Figure 6.32 D30Pr70L-PaDiMO projection of the fetlock.

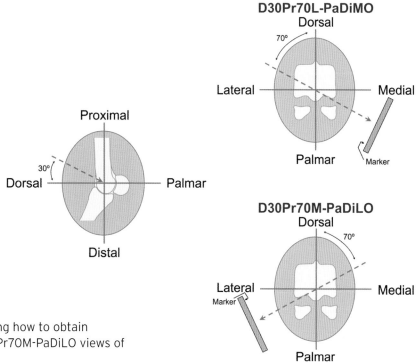

Figure 6.31 Diagram showing how to obtain D30Pr70L-PaDiMO and D30Pr70M-PaDiLO views of the fetlock.

Flexed dorsopalmar (flexed DPa) (Figs 6.33 and 6.34)

1. Flex the fetlock by placing the foot on a Hickman block, keeping the metacarpus/metatarsus vertical to the ground with gloved hands.
2. Place the plate in portrait orientation on the palmar side of the fetlock as close as possible to the limb.
3. Place a R/L marker on the lateral side of the plate.
4. Position the X-ray machine on the dorsal side of the foot.
5. Focus–film distance: 100 cm.
6. Use a horizontal X-ray beam.
7. Centre the X-ray beam at the level of the fetlock joint.
8. Collimate around the fetlock joint, including the distal third of the metacarpus/metatarsus.
9. Exposure guide: 70 kVp, 10 mAs.

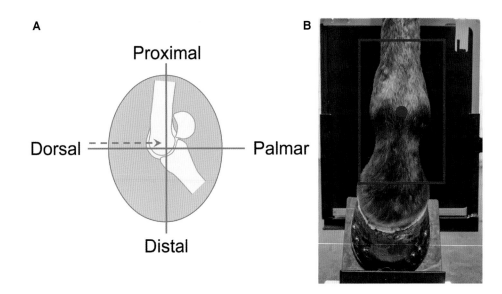

Figure 6.33 Diagram showing how to obtain a flexed DPa of the distal aspect of the metacarpus (A) and positioning to obtain the same view (B).

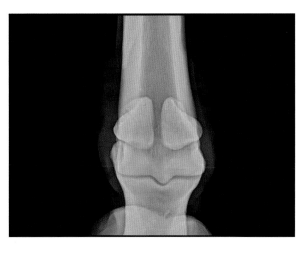

Figure 6.34 Flexed DPa projection of the distal aspect of the metacarpus.

Dorsodistal-palmaroproximal oblique (DDi-PaPrO) (Figs 6.35 and 6.36)

1. Position the foot on a flat block with the limb extended slightly forward relative to the horse.
2. Place the plate in portrait orientation parallel to the metacarpus/metatarsus on the palmar side of the fetlock, as close as possible to the limb.
3. Place a R/L marker on the lateral side of the plate.
4. Position the X-ray machine on the dorsal side of the limb, underneath the fetlock region.
5. Focus–film distance: 100 cm.
6. Angle the X-ray beam 15 degrees upward from the horizontal.
7. Centre the X-ray beam at the level of the fetlock joint.
8. Collimate around the fetlock joint, including the distal third of the metacarpus/metatarsus.
9. Exposure guide: 70 kVp, 10 mAs.

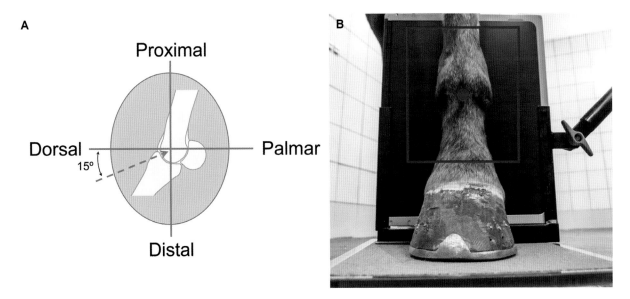

Figure 6.35 Diagram showing how to obtain a DDi-PaPrO of the distal aspect of the metacarpus (A) and positioning to obtain the same view (B).

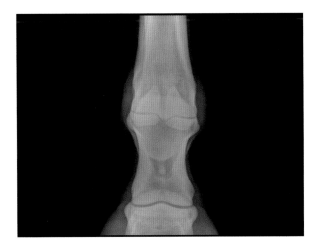

Figure 6.36 DDi-PaPrO projection of the distal aspect of the metacarpus.

CHAPTER 7

Metacarpus and metatarsus

Indications

Indications for performing radiographs of the metacarpus and metatarsus include:

- Lameness localized to this region by diagnostic analgesia (high four-point nerve block, lateral palmar block, high two-point block, deep branch of the lateral plantar nerve, subcarpal or subtarsal nerve blocks)
- Signs of trauma, such as wounds and swellings
- Bony swellings
- Pain on palpation.

Equipment

For a complete study of the metacarpus and metatarsus the following equipment is required:

- Portable X-ray machine
- Plate holder
- Radiation safety equipment: lead gowns, lead gloves and thyroid protectors.

Preparation

If necessary, brush or wash the area to reduce artefacts caused by dirt. Sedation of the patient is advised.

Radiographic protocol

A standard radiographic examination of the metacarpus/metatarsus usually includes four projections:

- Lateromedial (LM)
- Dorsopalmar (DPa)
- Dorso 45° lateral-palmaromedial oblique (D45L-PaMO) and dorso 45° medial-palmarolateral oblique (D45M-PaLO).

Additional projections for the distal metacarpus (already explained in Chapter 6):

- Flexed dorsopalmar (flexed DPa)
- Dorsodistal-palmaroproximal oblique (DDi-PaPrO).

Note: when radiographs of the metatarsus are obtained, the term palmar should be changed to plantar.

Lateromedial (LM) (Figs 7.1–7.4)

1. Stand the horse square with the cannon bone vertical to the ground in each direction and ensure that all limbs are equally weight-bearing.
2. Place the plate in portrait orientation on the medial side of the leg, as close as possible to the limb.
3. Place a R/L marker on the dorsal side of the plate.
4. Position the X-ray machine on the lateral side of the limb.
5. Focus–film distance: 100 cm.
6. Use a horizontal X-ray beam.
7. Align the beam perpendicular to the limb and the plate.
8. Centre the X-ray beam at the level of the metacarpus/metatarsus, midway between the fetlock and the carpus/tarsus.
9. Collimate around the area of interest.
10. Exposure guide: 60 kVp, 8 mAs.

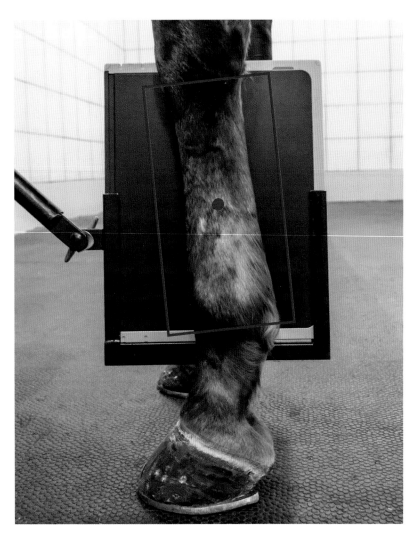

Figure 7.1 Positioning to obtain a LM view of the metacarpus.

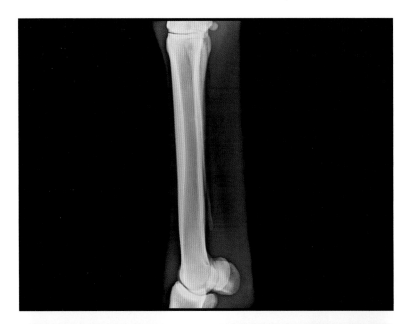

Figure 7.2 LM projection of the metacarpus.

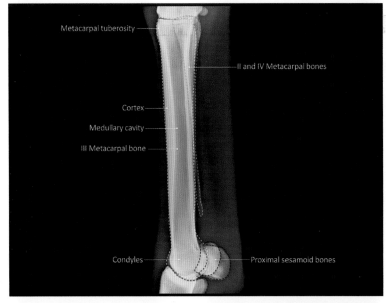

Figure 7.3 Radiographic anatomy of the LM projection of the metacarpus.

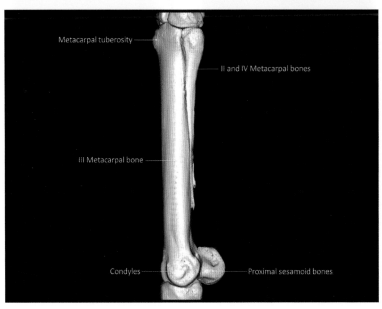

Figure 7.4 3D representation of the LM projection of the metacarpus.

Dorsopalmar (DPa) (Figs 7.5–7.8)

1. Stand the horse square with the cannon bone vertical to the ground in each direction and ensure that all limbs are equally weight-bearing.
2. Place the plate in portrait orientation on the palmar side of the leg, as close as possible to the limb.
3. Place a R/L marker on the lateral side of the plate.
4. Position the X-ray machine on the dorsal side of the limb.
5. Focus–film distance: 100 cm.
6. Use a horizontal X-ray beam.
7. Centre the X-ray beam at the level of the metacarpus/metatarsus, midway between the fetlock and the carpus/tarsus.
8. Collimate around the area of interest.
9. Exposure guide: 65 kVp, 10 mAs.

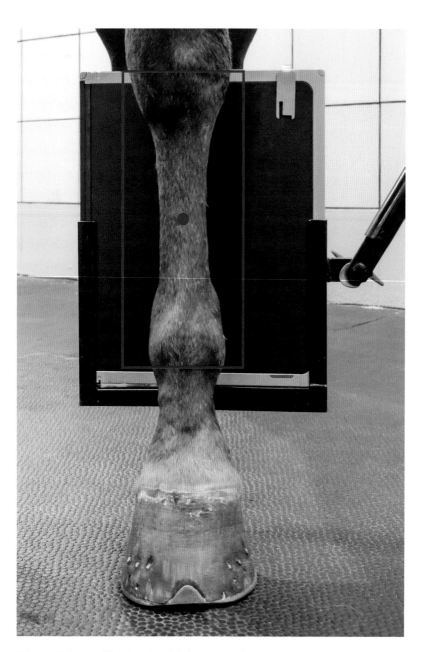

Figure 7.5 Positioning to obtain a DPa view of the metacarpus.

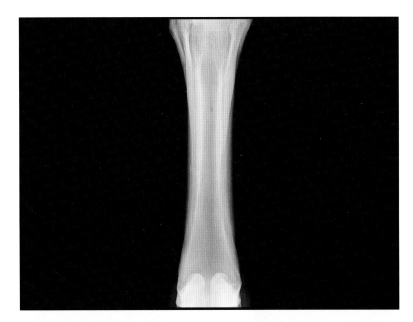

Figure 7.6 DPa projection of the metacarpus.

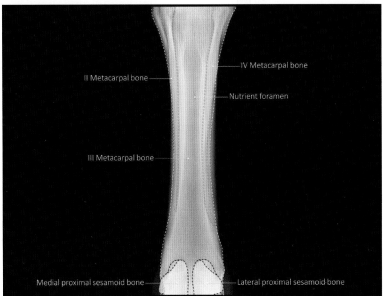

Figure 7.7 Radiographic anatomy of the DPa projection of the metacarpus.

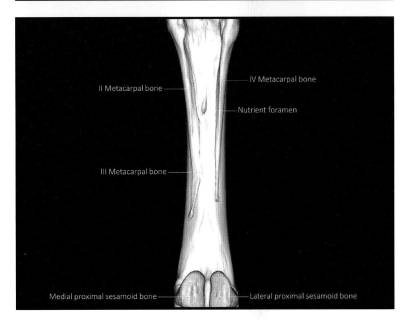

Figure 7.8 3D representation of the DPa projection of the metacarpus.

Dorso 45° lateral-palmaromedial oblique (D45L-PaMO) and dorso 45° medial-palmarolateral oblique (D45M-PaLO) (Figs 7.9–7.12)

1. Stand the horse square with the cannon bone vertical to the ground in each direction and ensure that all limbs are equally weight-bearing.
2. Place the plate in portrait orientation with a R/L marker on the lateral side.

   – D45L-PaMO: highlights the fourth metacarpal/metatarsal bone. The X-ray machine is positioned on the dorsolateral side of the leg, at a 45-degree angle from the sagittal plane of the limb. The plate is perpendicular to the X-ray beam on the palmaromedial side of the leg.
   – D45M-PaLO: highlights the second metacarpal/metatarsal bone. The X-ray machine is positioned on the dorsomedial side of the leg, at a 45-degree angle from the sagittal plane of the limb. The plate is perpendicular to the X-ray beam on the palmarolateral side of the leg.

3. Focus–film distance: 100 cm.
4. Use a horizontal X-ray beam.
5. Centre the X-ray beam at the level of the metacarpus/metatarsus, midway between the fetlock and the carpus/tarsus.
6. Collimate around the area of interest.
7. Exposure guide: 60 kVp, 8 mAs.
   Note: the D45M-PaLO can also be obtained as a Pa45L-DMO. The X-ray machine is positioned on the palmarolateral side of the leg, at a 45-degree angle from the sagittal plane of the limb. The plate is perpendicular to the X-ray beam on the dorsomedial side of the leg.

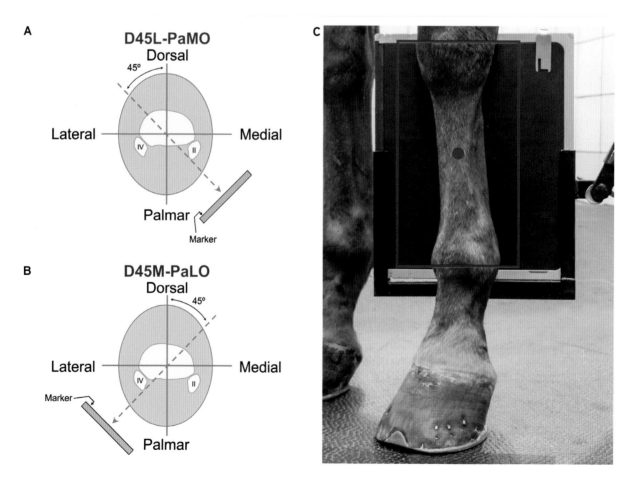

Figure 7.9 Diagram showing how to obtain D45L-PaMO (A) and D45M-PaLO (B) views of the metacarpus and positioning to obtain a D45L-PaMO view of the metacarpus (C).

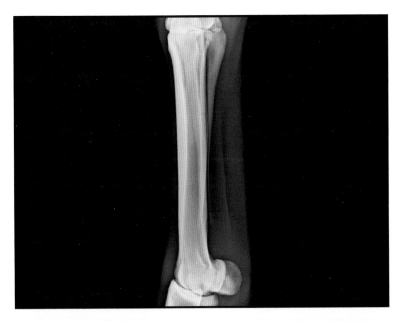

Figure 7.10 D45L-PaMO projection of the metacarpus.

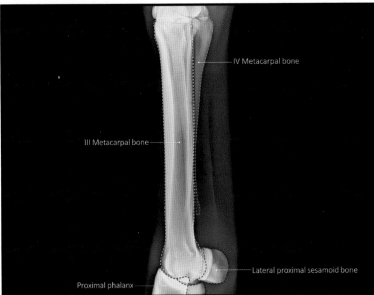

Figure 7.11 Radiographic anatomy of the D45L-PaMO projection of the metacarpus.

IV Metacarpal bone

III Metacarpal bone

Lateral proximal sesamoid bone

Proximal phalanx

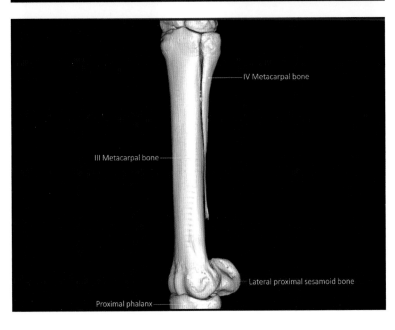

Figure 7.12 3D representation of the D45L-PaMO projection of the metacarpus.

IV Metacarpal bone

III Metacarpal bone

Lateral proximal sesamoid bone

Proximal phalanx

CHAPTER 8

Carpus

Indications

Carpal diseases are frequently described in young athletic horses, especially in racehorses, but carpal problems can also occur in older horses and in other disciplines.

Indications for performing radiographs of the carpus include:

- Lameness localized to the carpus by diagnostic analgesia (subcarpal, lateral palmar, high two-point, radial and ulnar nerve blocks, intercarpal joint block, radiocarpal joint block or carpal sheath block)
- Soft tissue swellings, including effusion of the carpal joints or the carpal sheath
- Signs of trauma, such as wounds or diffuse swelling
- Assessment of ossification status of the carpal bones in premature or dysmature foals
- Angular limb deformities of the carpal region
- As part of a pre-purchase and pre-sales examination.

Equipment

For a complete study of the carpus the following equipment is required:

- Portable X-ray machine
- Plate holder
- Radiation safety equipment: lead gowns, lead gloves and thyroid protectors.

Preparation

If necessary, brush or wash the area to reduce artefacts caused by dirt. Sedation of the patient is advised.

Radiographic protocol

A standard radiographic examination of the carpus usually includes at least five radiographs, although this may vary depending on the indication:

- Lateromedial (LM)
- Dorsopalmar (DPa)
- Dorso 45° lateral-palmaromedial oblique (D45L-PaMO)
- Dorso 45° medial-palmarolateral oblique (D45M-PaLO) or palmaro 45° lateral-dorsomedial oblique (Pa45L-DMO).

Additional projections:

- Flexed lateromedial (flexed LM)
- Dorso 85° proximal-dorsodistal oblique (D85Pr-DDiO) or 'skyline' view of the distal radius

- Dorso 55° proximal-dorsodistal oblique (D55Pr-DDiO) or 'skyline' view of the proximal row of carpal bones

- Dorso 35° proximal-dorsodistal oblique (D35Pr-DDiO) or 'skyline' view of the distal row of carpal bones.

Lateromedial (LM) (Figs 8.1–8.4)

1. Stand the horse square with the cannon bone vertical to the ground in each direction and ensure that all limbs are equally weight-bearing.
2. Place the plate in portrait orientation on the medial side of the carpus as close as possible to the limb.
3. Place a R/L marker on the dorsal side of the plate.
4. Position the X-ray machine on the lateral side of the limb.
5. Focus–film distance: 100 cm.
6. Use a horizontal X-ray beam perpendicularly aligned to the leg and plate.
7. Centre the X-ray beam at the level of the mid carpal joint.
8. Collimate around the carpus, including the proximal metacarpus.
9. Exposure guide: 70 kVp, 10 mAs.

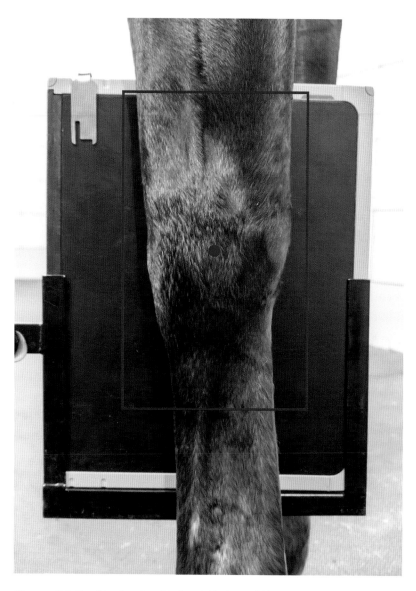

Figure 8.1 Positioning to obtain a LM view of the carpus.

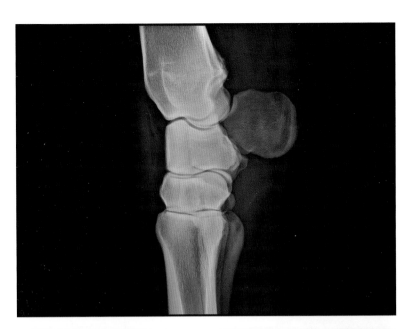

Figure 8.2 LM projection of the carpus.

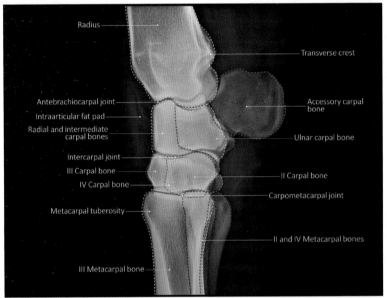

Figure 8.3 Radiographic anatomy of the LM projection of the carpus.

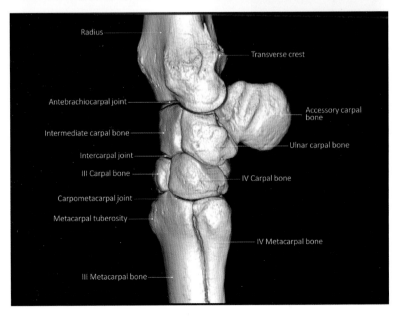

Figure 8.4 3D representation of the LM projection of the carpus.

Dorsopalmar (DPa) (Figs 8.5–8.8)

1. Stand the horse square with the cannon bone vertical to the ground in each direction and ensure that all limbs are equally weight-bearing.
2. Place the plate in portrait orientation on the palmar side of the joint as close as possible to the limb.
3. Place a R/L marker on the lateral side of the plate.
4. Position the X-ray machine on the dorsal side of the limb.
5. Focus–film distance: 100 cm.
6. Use a horizontal X-ray beam perpendicularly aligned to the leg and plate.
7. Centre the X-ray beam to the level of the mid carpal joint.
8. Collimate around the carpus, including the proximal metacarpus.
9. Exposure guide: 70 kVp, 10 mAs.

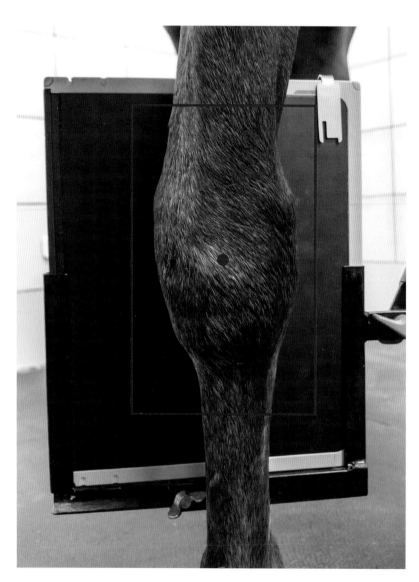

Figure 8.5 Positioning to obtain a DPa view of the carpus.

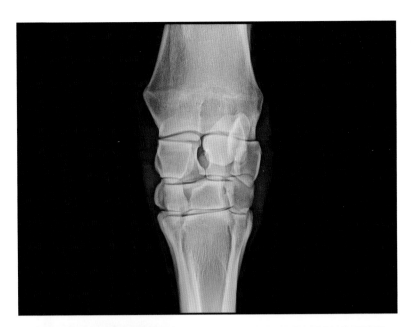

Figure 8.6 DPa projection of the carpus.

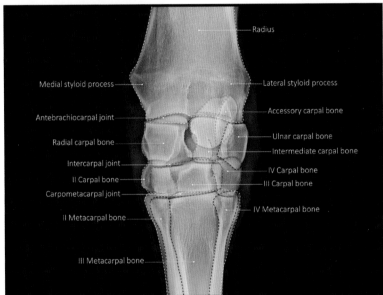

Figure 8.7 Radiographic anatomy of the DPa projection of the carpus.

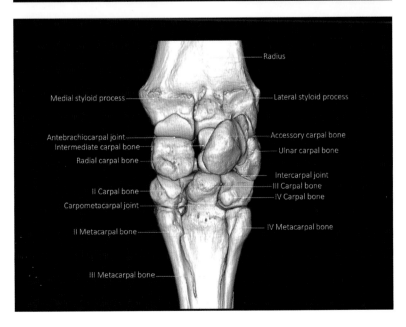

Figure 8.8 3D representation of the DPa projection of the carpus.

Dorso 45° lateral-palmaromedial oblique (D45L-PaMO) (Figs 8.9–8.12)

1. Stand the horse square with the cannon bone vertical to the ground in each direction and ensure that all limbs are equally weight-bearing.
2. Place the plate in portrait orientation palmaromedially to the joint as close as possible to the limb.
3. Place a R/L marker on the lateral side of the plate.
4. Position the X-ray machine dorsolaterally to the limb at a 45-degree angle from the sagittal plane of the limb.
5. Focus–film distance: 100 cm.
6. Use a horizontal X-ray beam.
7. Centre the X-ray beam at the level of the mid carpal joint.
8. Collimate around the carpus.
9. Exposure guide: 70 kVp, 10 mAs.

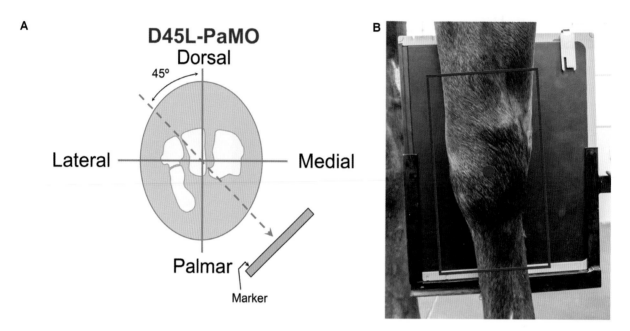

Figure 8.9 Diagram showing how to obtain D45L-PaMO view of the carpus (A) and positioning to obtain the same view (B).

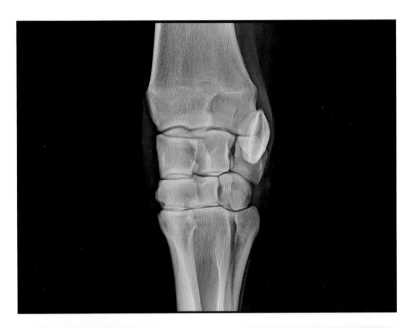

Figure 8.10 D45L-PaMO projection of the carpus.

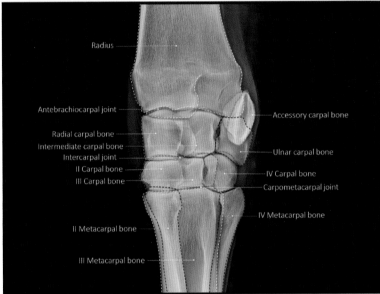

Figure 8.11 Radiographic anatomy of the D45L-PaMO projection of the carpus.

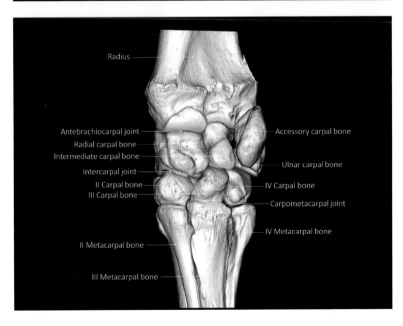

Figure 8.12 3D representation of the D45L-PaMO projection of the carpus.

Dorso 45° medial-palmarolateral oblique (D45M-PaLO) or palmaro 45° lateral-dorsomedial oblique (Pa45L-DMO) (Figs 8.13–8.16)

1. Stand the horse square with the cannon bone vertical to the ground in each direction and ensure that all limbs are equally weight-bearing.
2. Place the plate in portrait orientation with a R/L marker on its lateral side.

   – D45M-PaLO: the X-ray machine is positioned on the dorsomedial side of the joint, at a 45-degree angle from the sagittal plane of the limb. The plate is perpendicular to the X-ray beam on the palmarolateral side of the leg.
   – Pa45L-DMO: the X-ray machine is positioned on the palmarolateral side of the joint, at a 45-degree angle from the sagittal plane of the limb. The plate is perpendicular to the X-ray beam on the dorsomedial side of the leg.

3. Focus–film distance: 100 cm.
4. Use a horizontal X-ray beam.
5. Centre the X-ray beam at the level of the mid carpal joint.
6. Collimate around the carpus.
7. Exposure guide: 70 kVp, 10 mAs.

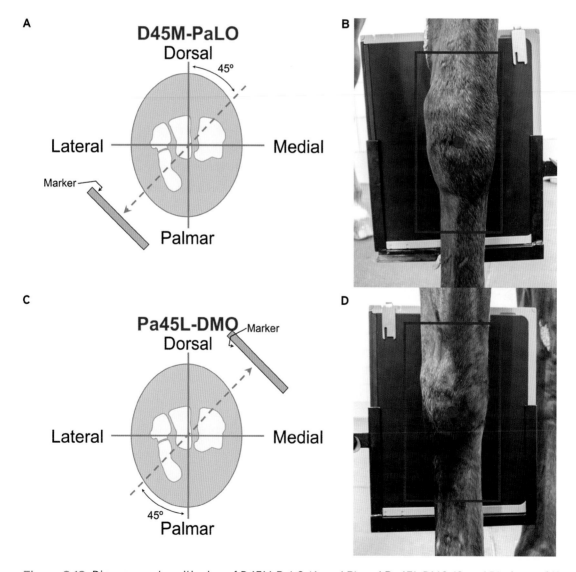

Figure 8.13 Diagram and positioning of D45M-PaLO (A and B) and Pa45L-DMO (C and D) views of the carpus.

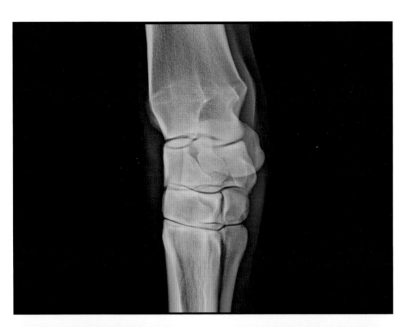

Figure 8.14 D45M-PaLO projection of the carpus.

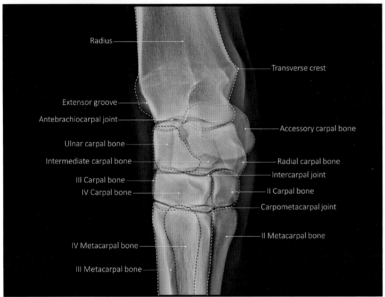

Figure 8.15 Radiographic anatomy of the D45M-PaLO projection of the carpus.

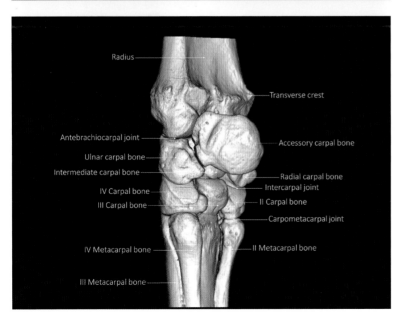

Figure 8.16 3D representation of the D45M-PaLO projection of the carpus.

Flexed lateromedial (flexed LM) (Figs 8.17–8.20)

1. Flex the carpus with gloved hands so that the metacarpus is horizontal.
2. Place the plate in landscape orientation on the medial side of the carpus as close as possible to the limb.
3. Place a R/L marker on the dorsal side of the plate.
4. Position the X-ray machine on the lateral side of the limb.
5. Focus–film distance: 100 cm
6. Use a horizontal X-ray beam perpendicularly aligned to the leg and plate.
7. Centre the X-ray beam at the level of the mid carpal joint.
8. Collimate around the carpus.
9. Exposure guide: 70 kVp, 10 mAs.

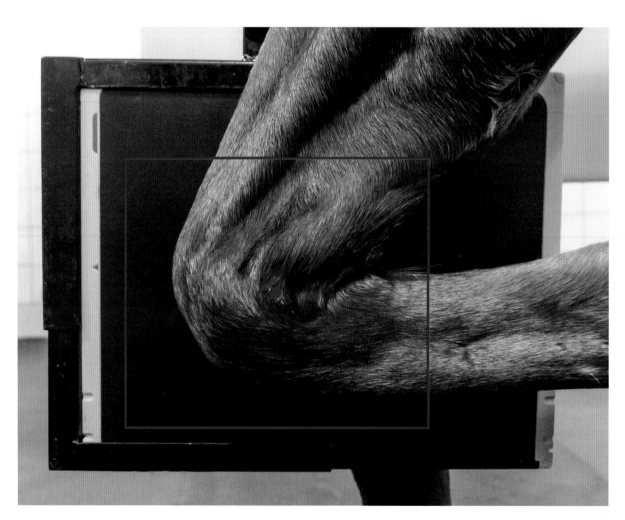

Figure 8.17 Positioning to obtain a flexed LM view of the carpus.

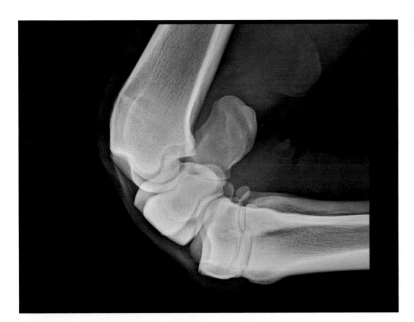

Figure 8.18 Flexed LM projection of the carpus.

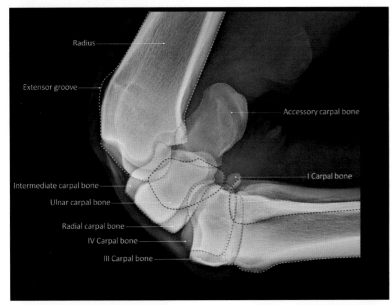

Figure 8.19 Radiographic anatomy of the flexed LM projection of the carpus.

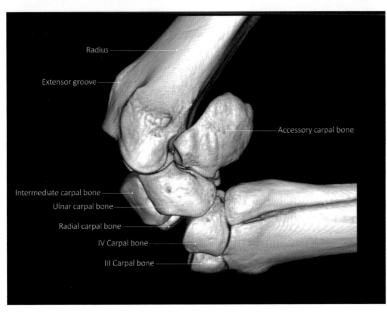

Figure 8.20 3D representation of the flexed LM projection of the carpus.

Dorso 85° proximal-dorsodistal oblique (D85Pr-DDiO) or 'skyline' view of the distal radius (Figs 8.21-8.24)

1. Flex the carpus with gloved hands so that the metacarpus is horizontal.
2. Place the plate in a horizontal position facing upwards under the metacarpus, extending beyond its dorsal border.
3. Place a R/L marker on the lateral side of the plate.
4. Position the X-ray machine on the cranial side of the limb above the carpal region.
5. Focus–film distance: 100 cm.
6. Angle the X-ray beam 85 degrees downward to the horizontal.
7. Centre the X-ray beam at the level of the cranial border of the distal radius.
8. Collimate around the cranial half of the distal radius.
9. Exposure guide: 65 kVp, 8 mAs.

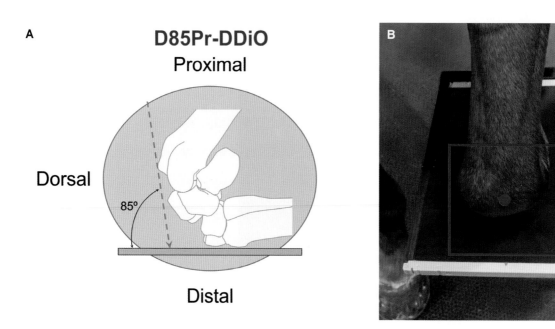

Figure 8.21 Diagram showing how to obtain D85Pr-DDiO view of the carpus (A) and positioning to obtain the same view (B).

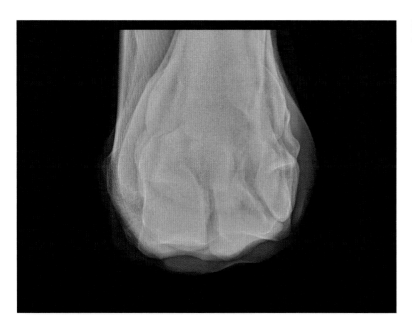

Figure 8.22 D85Pr-DDiO projection of the carpus.

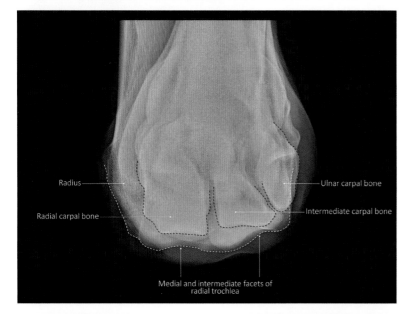

Figure 8.23 Radiographic anatomy of the D85Pr-DDiO projection of the carpus.

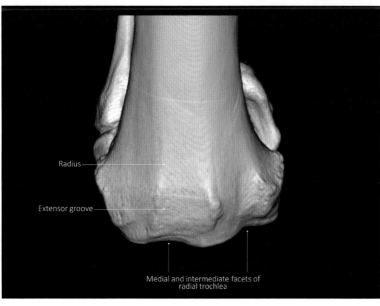

Figure 8.24 3D representation of the D85Pr-DDiO projection of the carpus.

Dorso 55° proximal-dorsodistal oblique (D55Pr-DDiO) or 'skyline' view of the proximal row of carpal bones (Figs 8.25-8.28)

1. Flex the carpus with gloved hands so that the metacarpus is horizontal.
2. Place the plate in a horizontal position facing upwards under the metacarpus, extending beyond its dorsal border.
3. Place a R/L marker on the lateral side of the plate.
4. Position the X-ray machine on the cranial side of the limb above the carpal region.
5. Focus–film distance: 100 cm.
6. Angle the X-ray beam 55 degrees downward to the horizontal.
7. Centre the X-ray beam at the level of the dorsal border of the proximal row of carpal bones.
8. Collimate around the dorsal half of the distal radius.
9. Exposure guide: 65 kVp, 8 mAs.

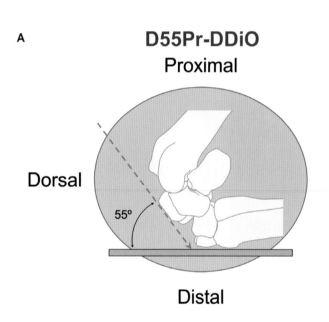
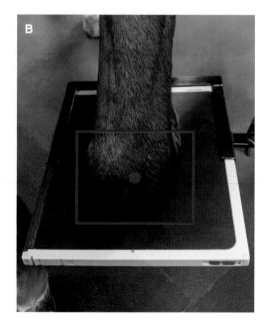

Figure 8.25 Diagram showing how to obtain D55Pr-DDiO view of the carpus (A) and positioning to obtain the same view (B).

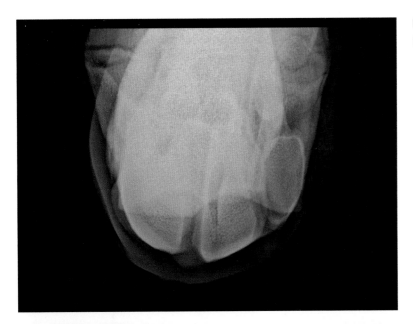

Figure 8.26 D55Pr-DDiO projection of the carpus.

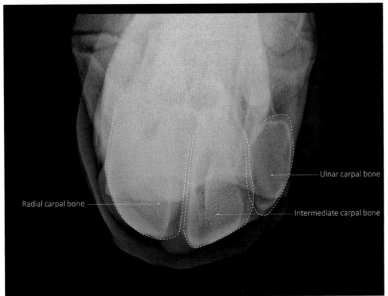

Figure 8.27 Radiographic anatomy of the D55Pr-DDiO projection of the carpus.

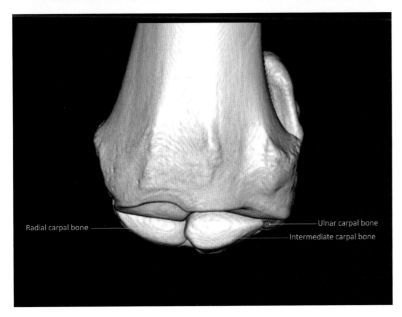

Figure 8.28 3D representation of the D55Pr-DDiO projection of the carpus.

Dorso 35° proximal-dorsodistal oblique (D35Pr-DDiO) or 'skyline' view of the distal row of carpal bones (Figs 8.29–8.32)

1. Flex the carpus with gloved hands so that the metacarpus is horizontal.
2. Place the plate in a horizontal position facing upwards under the metacarpus, extending beyond its dorsal border.
3. Place a R/L marker on the lateral side of the plate.
4. Position the X-ray machine on the cranial side of the limb above the carpal region.
5. Focus–film distance: 100 cm.
6. Angle the X-ray beam 35 degrees downward towards the horizontal.
7. Centre the X-ray beam at the level of the dorsal border of the distal row of carpal bones.
8. Collimate around the dorsal half of the distal radius.
9. Exposure guide: 65 kVp, 8 mAs.

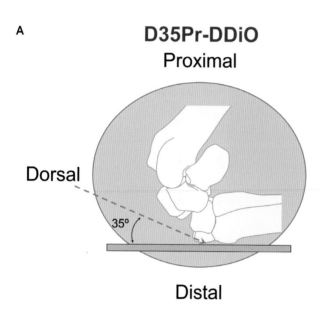

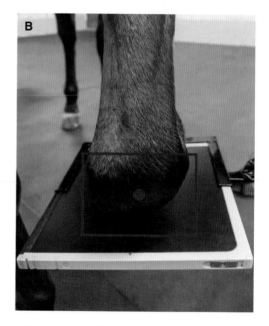

Figure 8.29 Diagram showing how to obtain D35Pr-DDiO view of the carpus (A) and positioning to obtain the same view (B).

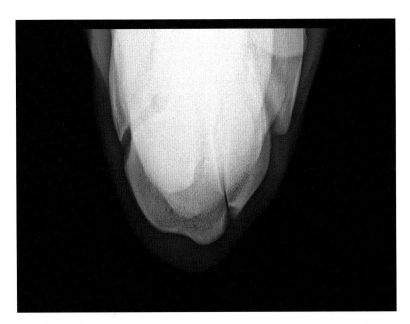

Figure 8.30 D35Pr-DDiO projection of the carpus.

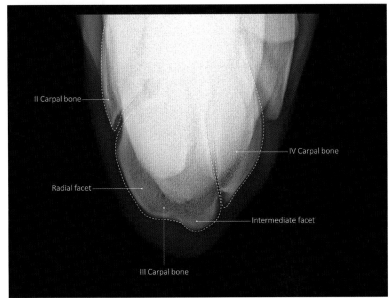

Figure 8.31 Radiographic anatomy of the D35Pr-DDiO projection of the carpus.

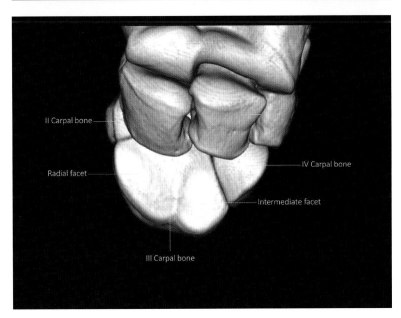

Figure 8.32 3D representation of the D35Pr-DDiO projection of the carpus.

CHAPTER 9

Elbow

Indications

Radiography of the elbow is not an everyday procedure for equine practitioners, but in certain circumstances it is an essential technique for an assessment of the bones in the elbow region, especially if a fracture is suspected.

Indications for performing radiographs of the elbow include:

- Clinical signs indicating a fracture in the region, e.g. a 'dropped' elbow appearance commonly associated with an olecranon fracture
- Signs of trauma, such as wounds and swellings
- Lameness localized to the elbow by diagnostic analgesia (humeroradial joint block).

Equipment

For a complete study of the elbow the following equipment is required:

- Portable X-ray machine is usually sufficient
- Large plates (35 × 43 cm) are recommended
- Plate holder
- Radiation safety equipment: lead gowns, lead gloves and thyroid protectors.

Preparation

If necessary, brush or wash the area to reduce artefacts caused by dirt. Sedation of the patient is advised.

Radiographic protocol

The standard radiographic examination of the elbow includes two radiographs:

- Mediolateral (ML)
- Craniocaudal (CrCd).

Additional oblique projections may be helpful in some cases:

- Cranio 45° medial-caudolateral oblique (Cr45M-CdLO).

Mediolateral (ML) (Figs 9.1–9.4)

1. Pull the leg forward with gloved hands until the radius is horizontally orientated to avoid the superimposition.
2. Place the plate in landscape orientation on the lateral side of the joint as close as possible to the limb.
3. Place a R/L marker on the dorsal side of the plate.
4. Position the X-ray machine on the other side of the horse, directing the beam underneath the base of the horse's neck.
5. Focus–film distance: 100 cm.
6. Use a horizontal X-ray beam perpendicularly aligned to the leg and plate.
7. Centre the X-ray beam on the area of interest. The elbow joint space can be palpated directly distal to the triceps muscle mass.
8. Collimate around the area of interest.
9. Exposure guide: 70 kVp, 20 mAs.

Note: some horses reject extending the leg and flexing the elbow, especially with painful conditions. In this case, take a lateromedial radiograph by not pulling the leg forward, but positioning the plate in portrait orientation between the leg and the trunk as far craniodorsally as possible. Position the X-ray machine lateral to the limb 100 cm away from the plate and use a horizontal X-ray beam perpendicularly aligned to the leg and plate. This view usually does not allow visualization of the whole area; however, it may result in a diagnostic view of the olecranon.

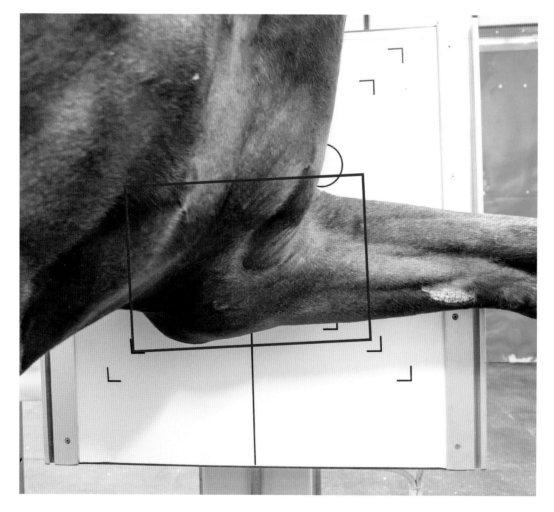

Figure 9.1 Positioning to obtain a ML view of the elbow.

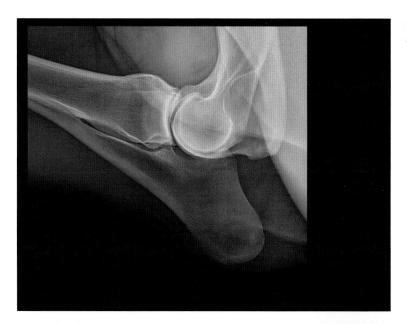

Figure 9.2 ML projection of the elbow.

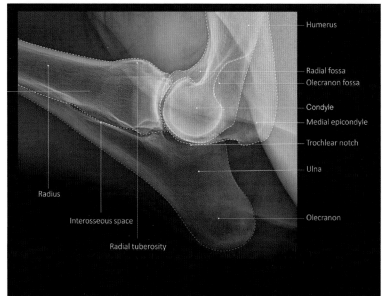

Figure 9.3 Radiographic anatomy of the ML projection of the elbow.

Humerus

Radial fossa
Olecranon fossa

Condyle
Medial epicondyle

Trochlear notch

Ulna

Olecranon

Radius

Interosseous space

Radial tuberosity

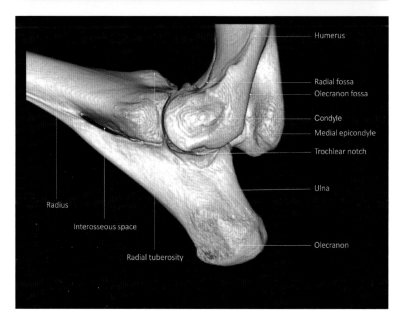

Figure 9.4 3D representation of the ML projection of the elbow.

Humerus

Radial fossa
Olecranon fossa

Condyle
Medial epicondyle

Trochlear notch

Ulna

Olecranon

Radius

Interosseous space

Radial tuberosity

Craniocaudal (CrCd) (Figs 9.5–9.8)

1. Position the horse as equally weight-bearing as possible; this may be challenging in horses with painful conditions.
2. Slight outward rotation of the limb is often helpful.
3. Place the plate on the caudal aspect of the elbow. This requires pushing the plate in and up as much as possible. Tilt the plate to increase the field of view.
4. Place a R/L marker on the lateral side of the plate.
5. Position the X-ray machine cranial to the limb.
6. Focus–film distance: 100 cm.
7. Use a horizontal X-ray beam perpendicularly aligned to the leg and plate.
8. Centre the X-ray beam on the area of interest.
9. Collimate around the area of interest.
10. Exposure guide: 80 kVp, 20 mAs.

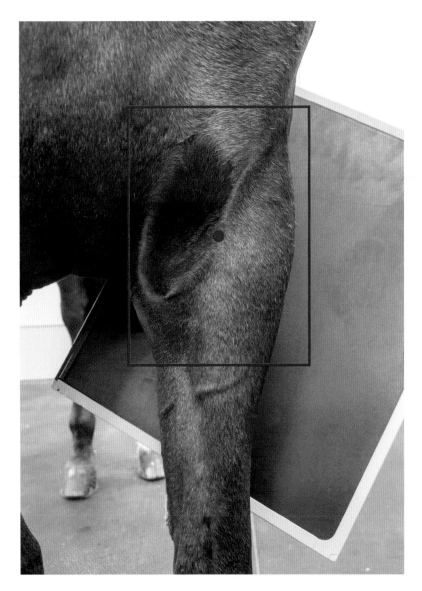

Figure 9.5 Positioning to obtain a CrCd view of the elbow.

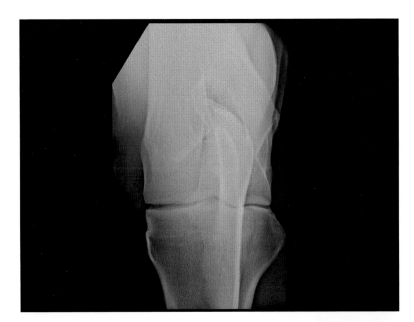

Figure 9.6 CrCd projection of the elbow.

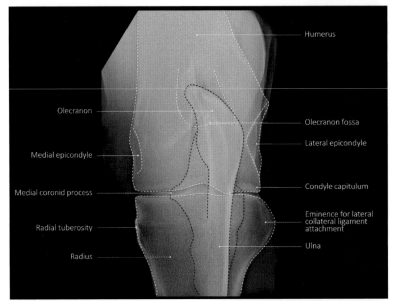

Figure 9.7 Radiographic anatomy of the CrCd projection of the elbow.

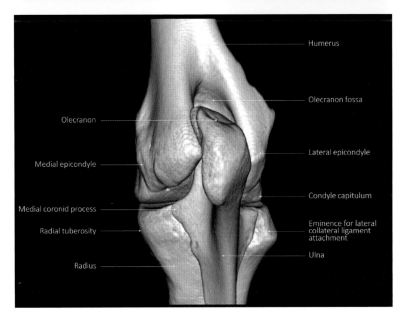

Figure 9.8 3D representation of the CrCd projection of the elbow.

Cranio 45° medial-caudolateral oblique (Cr45M-CdLO) (Figs 9.9–9.12)

1. Position the horse as equally weight-bearing as possible; this may be challenging in horses with painful conditions.
2. Place the plate in portrait orientation on the caudolateral side of the joint, as close as possible to the limb.
3. Place a R/L marker on the lateral side of the plate.
4. Position the X-ray machine craniomedially to the limb at a 45-degree angle to the sagittal plane of the trunk.
5. Focus–film distance: 100 cm.
6. Use a horizontal X-ray beam.
7. Centre the X-ray beam on the elbow joint.
8. Collimate around the elbow.
9. Exposure guide: 80 kVp, 20 mAs.

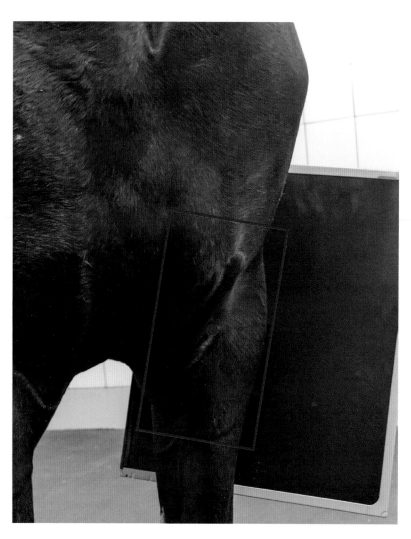

Figure 9.9 Positioning to obtain a Cr45M-CdLO view of the elbow.

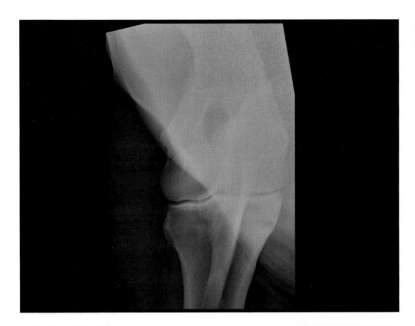

Figure 9.10 Cr45M-CdLO projection of the elbow.

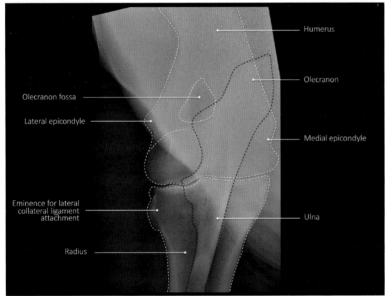

Figure 9.11 Radiographic anatomy of the Cr45M-CdLO projection of the elbow.

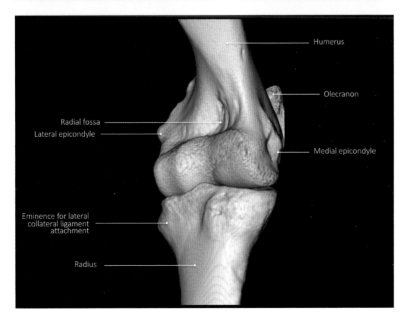

Figure 9.12 3D representation of the Cr45M-CdLO projection of the elbow.

CHAPTER 10

Shoulder

Indications

Radiography of the shoulder is not a routine procedure, largely because shoulder lameness is relatively uncommon. However, quality shoulder radiographs are useful for certain conditions affecting the shoulder, including fractures, osteochondrosis, osteoarthritis or shoulder dysplasia.

Indications for performing radiographs of the shoulder include:

- Lameness localized to the shoulder by diagnostic analgesia (scapulohumeral joint block)
- Soft tissue and bony swellings
- Signs of trauma
- Lameness in Shetland ponies that cannot be attributed to other regions.

Equipment

For a complete study of the shoulder the following equipment is required:

- High-output X-ray generator
- Large plates (35 × 43 cm)
- Plate holder: ceiling/wall-mounted
- Grid: should be used to reduce scatter and improve image quality
- Radiation safety equipment: lead gowns, lead gloves and thyroid protectors.

Preparation

If necessary, brush or wash the area to reduce artefacts caused by dirt. Sedation of the patient is advised.

Radiographic protocol

A standard radiographic examination of the shoulder usually includes a minimum of two radiographs, although this may vary depending on the suspected disease:

- Mediolateral (ML)
- Cranio 45° medial-caudolateral oblique (Cr45M-CdLO).

Additional projections

- Cranioproximal-craniodistal oblique (CrPr-CrDiO) or 'skyline' view of the proximal aspect of the humerus.

Mediolateral (ML) (Figs 10.1–10.4)

1. Pull the leg forward with gloved hands as far as possible to prevent superimposition of the contralateral shoulder and raise the head and neck to avoid superimposition of the cervical spine over the distal aspect of the scapula. Ideally, the trachea would be superimposed over the shoulder joint to increase contrast.
2. Place the plate in portrait orientation on the lateral side of the shoulder.
3. Place a R/L marker on the dorsal side of the plate.
4. Position the X-ray machine on the other side of the horse. The X-ray beam will be directed under the neck of the horse.
5. Focus–film distance: 100 cm. If a grid is used, adjust the focus–film distance to the distance specified for the grid.
6. Use a horizontal X-ray beam perpendicularly aligned to the leg and plate.
7. Centre the X-ray beam on the trachea, approximately 5–10 cm in front of the distal end of the scapular spine of the contralateral limb.
8. Collimate tightly around the shoulder to reduce scatter.
9. Exposure guide: 90 kVp, 40 mAs.

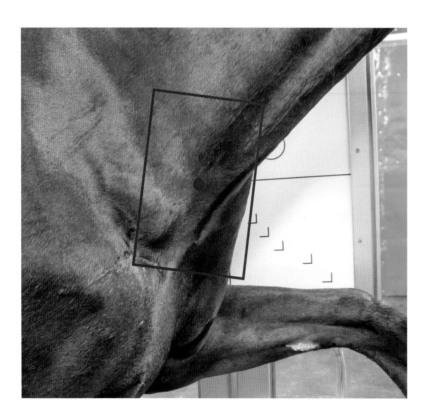

Figure 10.1 Positioning to obtain a ML view of the shoulder.

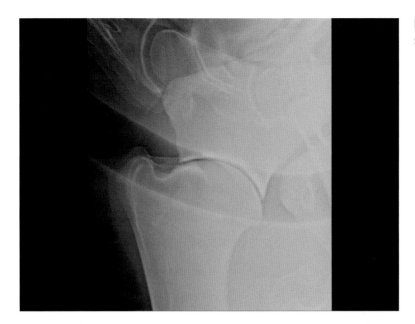

Figure 10.2 ML projection of the shoulder.

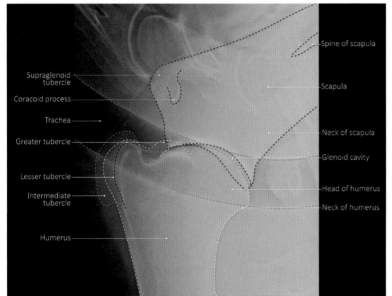

Figure 10.3 Radiographic anatomy of the ML projection of the shoulder.

Figure 10.4 3D representation of the ML projection of the shoulder.

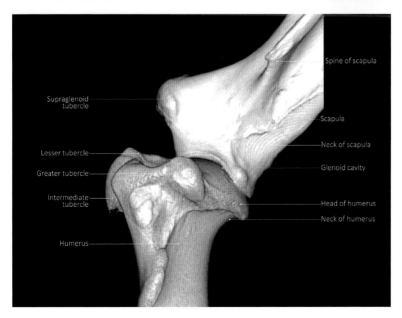

Cranio 45° medial-caudolateral oblique (Cr45M-CdLO) (Figs 10.5–10.8)

1. Pull the leg forward with gloved hands.
2. Place the plate in portrait orientation on the caudolateral side of the joint, as close as possible to the limb.
3. Place a R/L marker on the lateral side of the plate.
4. Position the X-ray machine craniomedially to the limb at a 45-degree angle to the sagittal plane of the limb.
5. Focus–film distance: 100 cm. If a grid is used, adjust the focus–film distance to the distance specified for the grid.
6. Use a horizontal X-ray beam.
7. Centre the X-ray beam on the greater tubercle of the humerus (easily palpated).
8. Collimate tightly around the shoulder to reduce scatter.
9. Exposure guide: 75 kVp, 30 mAs.

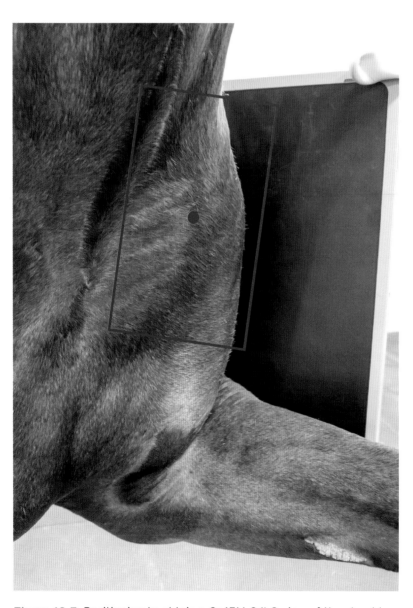

Figure 10.5 Positioning to obtain a Cr45M-CdLO view of the shoulder.

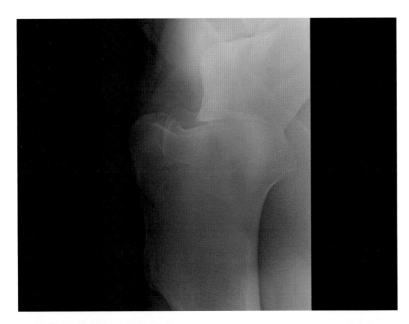

Figure 10.6 Cr45M-CdLO projection of the shoulder.

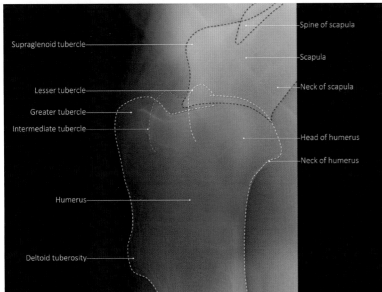

Figure 10.7 Radiographic anatomy of the Cr45M-CdLO projection of the shoulder.

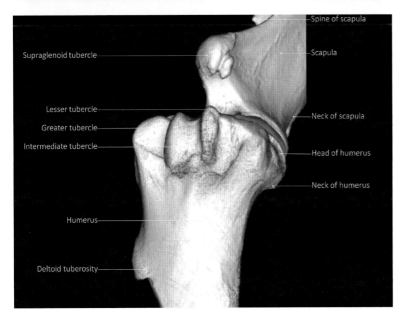

Figure 10.8 3D representation of the Cr45M-CdLO projection of the shoulder.

Cranioproximal-craniodistal oblique (CrPr-CrDiO) or 'skyline' view of the proximal aspect of the humerus (Figs 10.9–10.12)

1. Flex the carpus and elbow joints with gloved hands and bend the horse's neck away from the side of interest. Slight outward rotation of the limb is usually helpful.
2. Place the plate in a horizontal position facing upwards distal to the shoulder.
3. Place a R/L marker on the lateral side of the plate.
4. Position the X-ray machine above the shoulder. A 100 cm focus–film distance is usually not possible since the X-ray machine cannot be positioned high enough in relation to the humerus.
5. Use a vertical X-ray beam.
6. Centre the X-ray beam on the humeral tubercles.
7. Collimate around the shoulder.
8. Exposure guide: 75 kVp, 30 mAs.

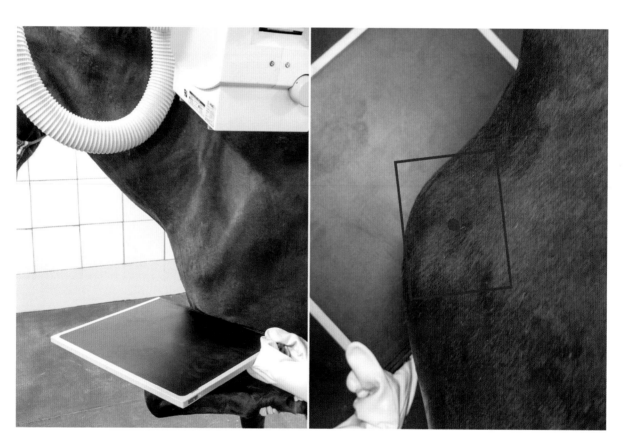

Figure 10.9 Positioning to obtain a CrPr-CrDiO view of the shoulder.

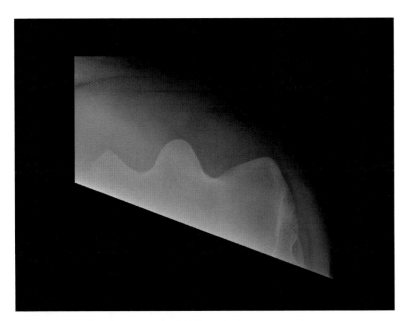

Figure 10.10 CrPr-CrDiO projection of the shoulder.

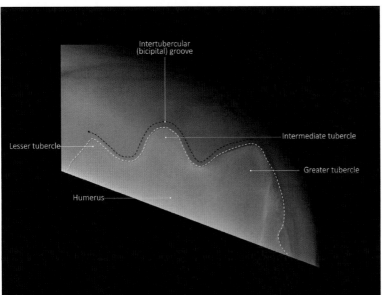

Figure 10.11 Radiographic anatomy of the CrPr-CrDiO projection of the shoulder.

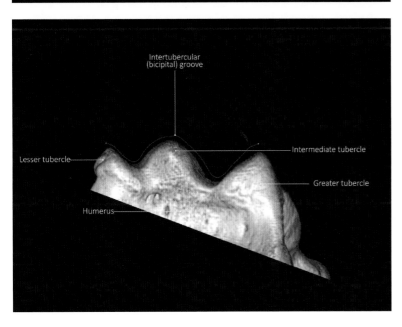

Figure 10.12 3D representation of the CrPr-CrDiO projection of the shoulder.

CHAPTER 11

Tarsus

Indications

Disorders of the tarsus are a common cause of hind limb lameness in the horse and therefore radiography of the tarsal region is a routine procedure in equine practice.

Indications for performing radiographs of the tarsus include:

- Lameness localized to the tarsus by diagnostic analgesia, including subtarsal, deep branch of the lateral plantar nerve, peroneal and tibial nerve blocks, tarsocrural joint block, distal intertarsal joint block, tarsometatarsal joint block or tarsal sheath block
- Soft tissue swellings, including effusion of synovial structures, e.g. the tarsocrural joint or the tarsal sheath
- Signs of trauma, such as wounds or diffuse swellings
- Assessment of tarsal bone ossification in premature or dysmature foals
- Angular limb deformities of the tarsal region
- As part of a pre-purchase or pre-sales examination.

Equipment

For a complete study of the tarsus the following equipment is required:

- Portable X-ray machine
- Plate holder
- Radiation safety equipment: lead gowns, lead gloves and thyroid protectors.

Preparation

If necessary, brush or wash the area to reduce artefacts caused by dirt. Sedation of the patient is advised.

Radiographic protocol

A standard radiographic examination of the tarsus usually includes at least four radiographs, although this may vary depending on the indication:

- Lateromedial (LM)
- Dorsoplantar (DPl)
- Dorso 45° lateral-plantaromedial oblique (D45L-PlMO)
- Dorso 45° medial-plantarolateral oblique (D45M-PlLO) or plantaro 45° lateral-dorsomedial oblique (Pl45L-DMO).

Additional projections:

- Flexed lateromedial (flexed LM)
- Flexed dorsoplantar (flexed DPl) or 'skyline' view of the tuber calcanei/sustentaculum tali.

Lateromedial (LM) (Figs 11.1–11.4)

1. Stand the horse square with the cannon bone vertical to the ground in each direction, and ensure all limbs are equally weight-bearing.
2. Place the plate in portrait orientation on the medial side of the tarsus as close as possible to the limb.
3. Place a R/L marker on the dorsal side of the plate.
4. Position the X-ray machine on the lateral side of the limb.
5. Focus–film distance: 100 cm.
6. Use a horizontal X-ray beam perpendicularly aligned to the tarsus. Beware not to use the foot to align your X-ray beam since many horses stand 'toe out'.
7. Centring: the distal intertarsal joint and the tarsometatarsal joint slope downward from lateral to medial and there are two methods to achieve a good view through these joint spaces:

   – Centre the horizontal X-ray beam at the level of the lateral malleolus of the tibia. Due to the divergent nature of the X-ray beam the X-rays will have a 3–5-degree angle at the level of the distal joints.
   – Centre on distal intertarsal and tarsometatarsal joints (about 10 cm below the point of the hock or 2 cm above the head of the fourth metatarsal bone) and angle the X-ray beam 5 degrees downward from the horizontal.

8. Collimate around the tarsus, including the proximal metatarsus and the tuber calcanei.
9. Exposure guide: 70 kVp, 10 mAs.

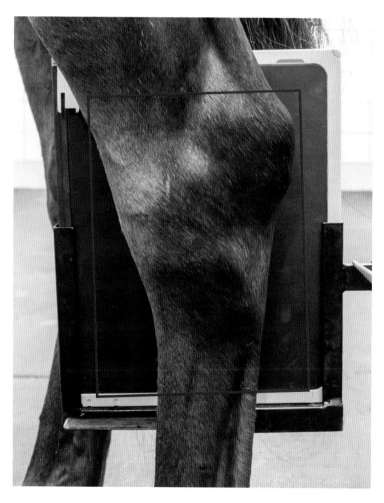

Figure 11.1 Positioning to obtain a LM view of the tarsus.

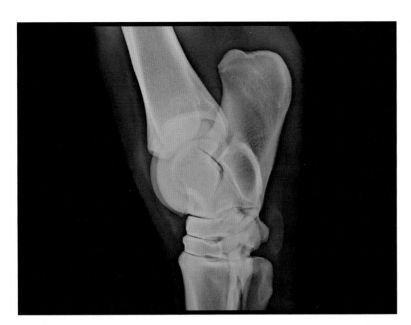

Figure 11.2 LM projection of the tarsus.

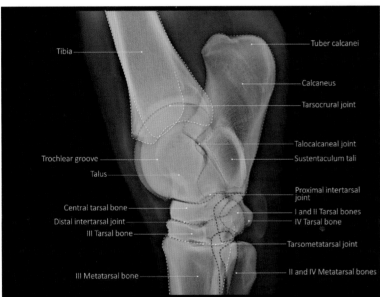

Figure 11.3 Radiographic anatomy of the LM projection of the tarsus.

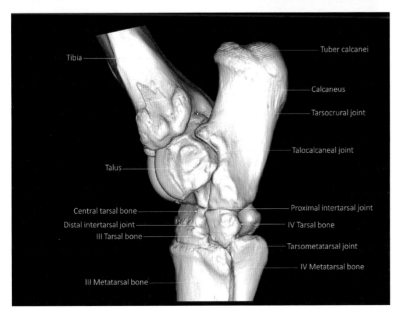

Figure 11.4 3D representation of the LM projection of the tarsus.

Dorsoplantar (DPl) (Figs 11.5–11.8)

1. Stand the horse square with the cannon bone vertical to the ground in each direction, and ensure all limbs are equally weight-bearing.
2. Place the plate in portrait orientation on the plantar side of the joint as close as possible to the limb.
3. Place a R/L marker on the lateral side of the plate.
4. Position the X-ray machine on the dorsal side of the limb.
5. Focus–film distance: 100 cm.
6. Use a horizontal X-ray beam perpendicularly aligned to the leg. In some horses, it is necessary to angle 5–10 degrees downward from horizontal to see through the joint spaces.
7. Centre the X-ray beam at the level of the distal intertarsal joint (about 10 cm below the point of the hock or 2 cm above the head of the fourth metatarsal bone).
8. Collimate around the tarsus.
9. Exposure guide: 70 kVp, 10 mAs.

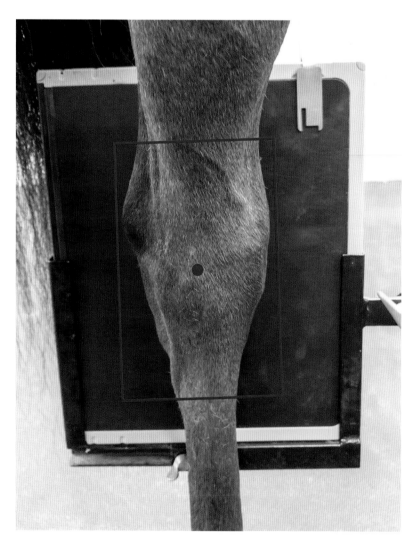

Figure 11.5 Positioning to obtain a DPl view of the tarsus.

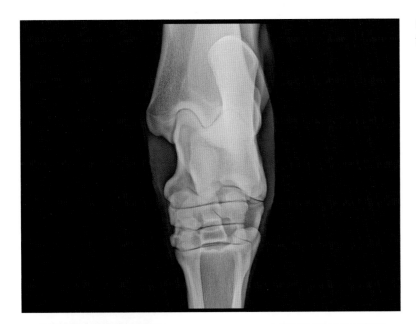

Figure 11.6 DPI projection of the tarsus.

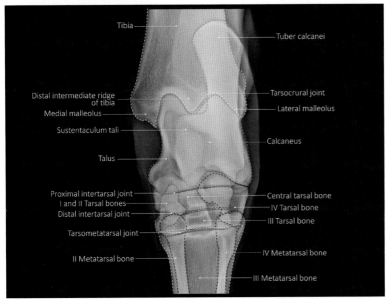

Figure 11.7 Radiographic anatomy of the DPI projection of the tarsus.

Tibia

Tuber calcanei

Distal intermediate ridge of tibia

Tarsocrural joint

Medial malleolus

Lateral malleolus

Sustentaculum tali

Talus

Calcaneus

Proximal intertarsal joint

Central tarsal bone

I and II Tarsal bones

IV Tarsal bone

Distal intertarsal joint

III Tarsal bone

Tarsometatarsal joint

II Metatarsal bone

IV Metatarsal bone

III Metatarsal bone

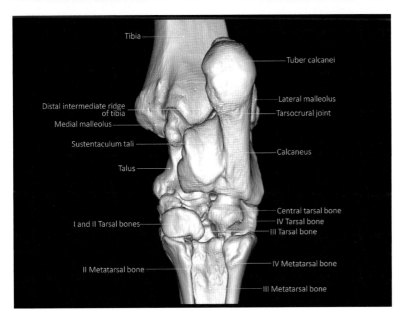

Figure 11.8 3D representation of the DPI projection of the tarsus.

Tibia

Tuber calcanei

Distal intermediate ridge of tibia

Lateral malleolus

Medial malleolus

Tarsocrural joint

Sustentaculum tali

Talus

Calcaneus

Central tarsal bone

I and II Tarsal bones

IV Tarsal bone

III Tarsal bone

II Metatarsal bone

IV Metatarsal bone

III Metatarsal bone

Dorso 45° lateral-plantaromedial oblique (D45L-PIMO) (Figs 11.9–11.12)

1. Stand the horse square with the cannon bone vertical to the ground in each direction, and ensure all limbs are equally weight-bearing.
2. Place the plate in portrait orientation plantaromedially to the joint as close as possible to the limb.
3. Place a R/L marker on the lateral side of the plate.
4. Position the X-ray machine dorsolaterally to the limb at a 45-degree angle from the sagittal plane of the limb.
5. Focus–film distance: 100 cm.
6. Use a horizontal X-ray beam.
7. Centre the X-ray beam at the level of the distal intertarsal joint (about 10 cm below the point of the hock or 2 cm above the head of the fourth metatarsal bone).
8. Collimate around the tarsus.
9. Exposure guide: 70 kVp, 10 mAs.

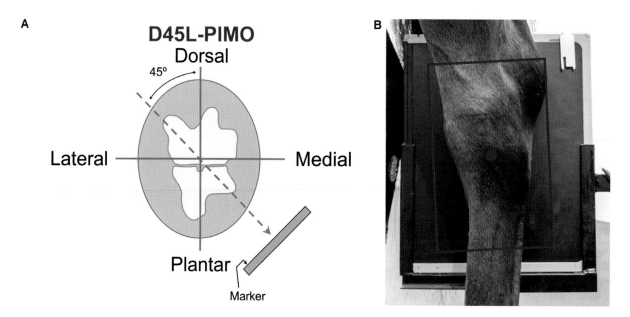

Figure 11.9 Diagram showing how to obtain a D45L-PIMO view of the tarsus (A) and positioning to obtain the same view (B).

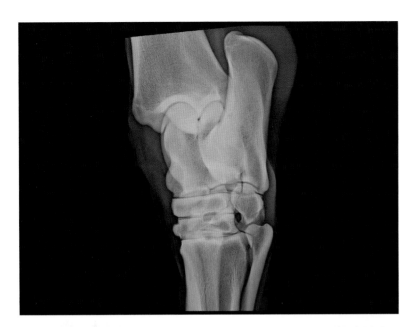

Figure 11.10 D45L-PlMO projection of the tarsus.

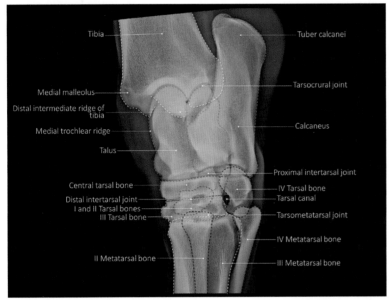

Figure 11.11 Radiographic anatomy of the D45L-PlMO projection of the tarsus.

Tibia

Medial malleolus

Distal intermediate ridge of tibia

Medial trochlear ridge

Talus

Central tarsal bone

Distal intertarsal joint

I and II Tarsal bones

III Tarsal bone

II Metatarsal bone

Tuber calcanei

Tarsocrural joint

Calcaneus

Proximal intertarsal joint

IV Tarsal bone

Tarsal canal

Tarsometatarsal joint

IV Metatarsal bone

III Metatarsal bone

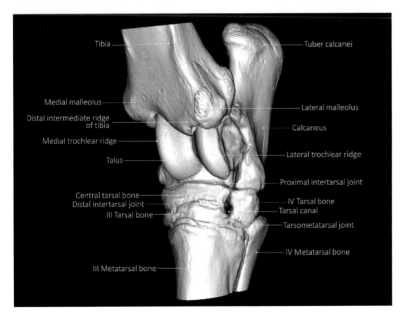

Figure 11.12 3D representation of the D45L-PlMO projection of the tarsus.

Tibia

Medial malleolus

Distal intermediate ridge of tibia

Medial trochlear ridge

Talus

Central tarsal bone

Distal intertarsal joint

III Tarsal bone

III Metatarsal bone

Tuber calcanei

Lateral malleolus

Calcaneus

Lateral trochlear ridge

Proximal intertarsal joint

IV Tarsal bone

Tarsal canal

Tarsometatarsal joint

IV Metatarsal bone

Dorso 45° medial-plantarolateral oblique (D45M-PlLO) or plantaro 45° lateral-dorsomedial oblique (Pl45L-DMO) (Figs 11.13–11.16)

1. Stand the horse square with the cannon bone vertical to the ground in each direction, and ensure all limbs are equally weight-bearing.
2. Place the plate in portrait orientation with a R/L marker on its lateral side.

   – D45M-PlLO: the X-ray machine is positioned on the dorsomedial side of the joint, at a 45-degree angle from the sagittal plane of the limb. The plate is perpendicular to the X-ray beam on the plantarolateral side of the leg.

   – Pl45L-DMO: the X-ray machine is positioned on the plantarolateral side of the joint, at a 45-degree angle from the sagittal plane of the limb. The plate is perpendicular to the X-ray beam on the dorsomedial side of the leg.

3. Focus–film distance: 100 cm.
4. Use a horizontal X-ray beam.
5. Centre the X-ray beam at the level of the distal intertarsal joint (about 10 cm below the point of the hock or 2 cm above the head of the fourth metatarsal bone).
6. Collimate around the tarsus.
7. Exposure guide: 70 kVp, 10 mAs.

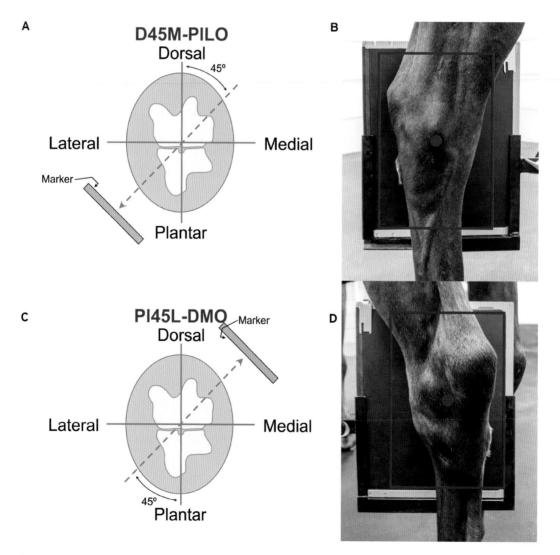

Figure 11.13 Diagram and positioning of D45M-PlLO (A and B) and Pl45L-DMO (C and D) views of the tarsus.

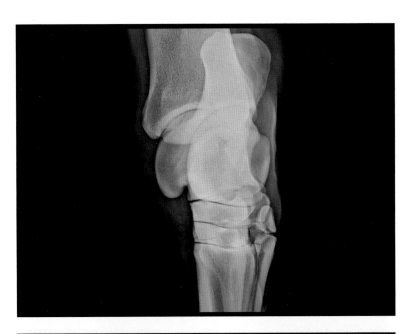

Figure 11.14 D45M-PILO projection of the tarsus.

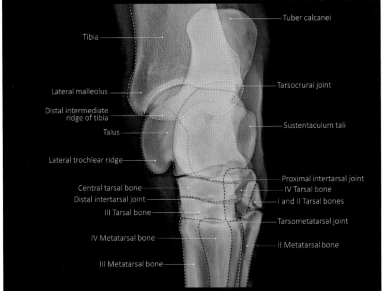

Figure 11.15 Radiographic anatomy of the D45M-PILO projection of the tarsus.

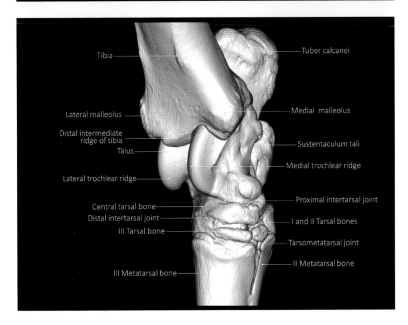

Figure 11.16 3D representation of the D45M-PILO projection of the tarsus.

Flexed lateromedial (flexed LM) (Figs 11.17–11.20)

1. Flex the tarsus with gloved hands so that the metatarsus is at about 30 degrees to the ground.
2. Place the plate in landscape orientation on the medial side of the tarsus as close as possible to the limb.
3. Place a R/L marker on the dorsal side of the plate.
4. Position the X-ray machine on the lateral side of the limb.
5. Focus–film distance: 100 cm.
6. Use a horizontal X-ray beam perpendicularly aligned to the leg and plate.
7. Centre the X-ray beam dorsal to the calcaneus.
8. Collimate around the tarsus.
9. Exposure guide: 70 kVp, 10 mAs.

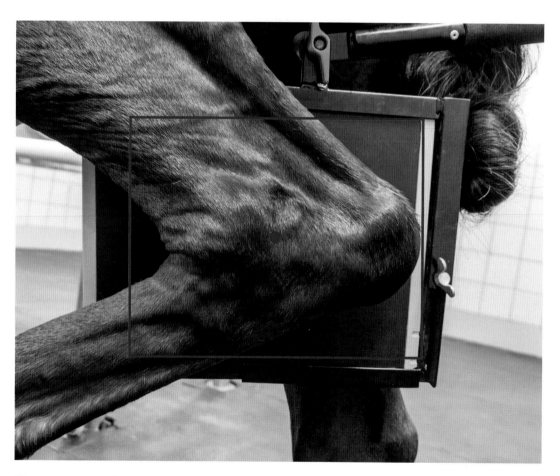

Figure 11.17 Positioning to obtain a flexed LM view of the tarsus.

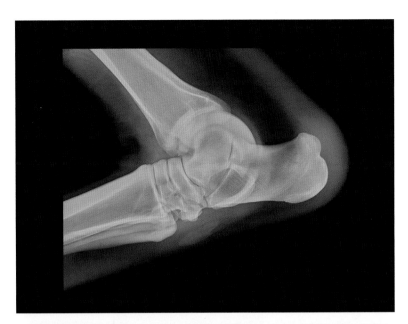

Figure 11.18 Flexed LM projection of the tarsus.

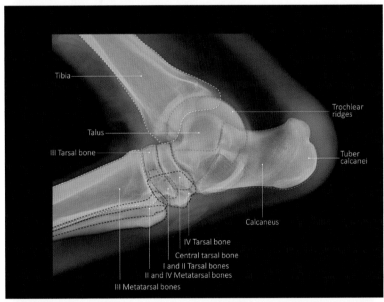

Figure 11.19 Radiographic anatomy of the flexed LM projection of the tarsus.

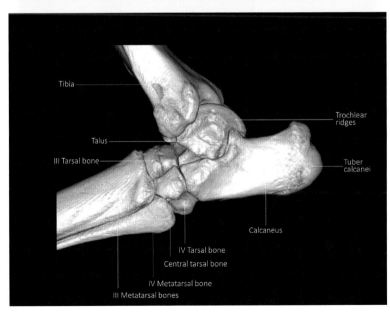

Figure 11.20 3D representation of the flexed LM projection of the tarsus.

Flexed dorsoplantar (flexed DPI) or 'skyline' view of the tuber calcanei/ sustentaculum tali (Figs 11.21–11.24)

1. Flex the tarsus with gloved hands so that the metatarsus is at about 30 degrees to the ground. The tarsus should be held as far behind the horse as possible.
2. Place the plate in a horizontal position facing upwards under the metatarsus and extending beyond its proximal border.
3. Place a R/L marker on the lateral side of the plate.
4. Position the X-ray machine caudal to the limb and above the tarsal region.
5. Focus–film distance: 100 cm.
6. Angle the X-ray beam downwards as close to the vertical as possible.
7. Centre the X-ray beam at the level of the calcaneus.
8. Collimate around the area of interest.
9. Exposure guide: 65 kVp, 10 mAs.

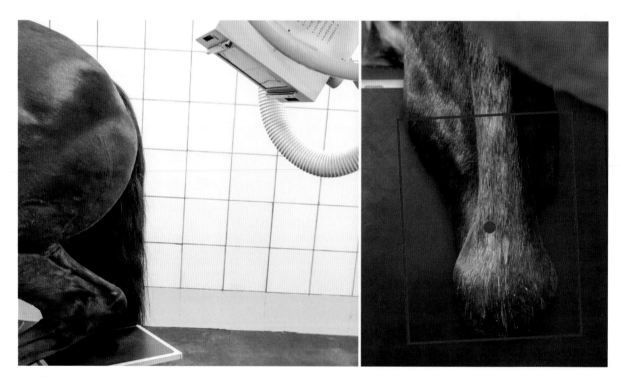

Figure 11.21 Positioning to obtain a flexed DPI view of the tarsus.

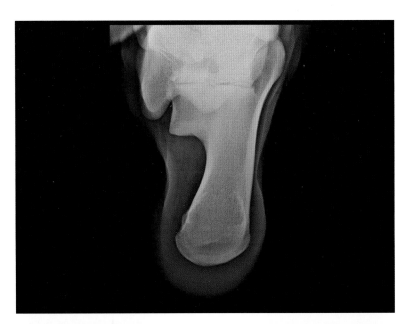

Figure 11.22 Flexed DPI projection of the tarsus.

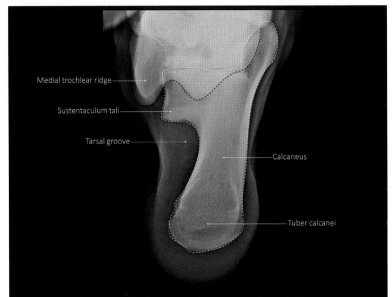

Figure 11.23 Radiographic anatomy of the flexed DPI projection of the tarsus.

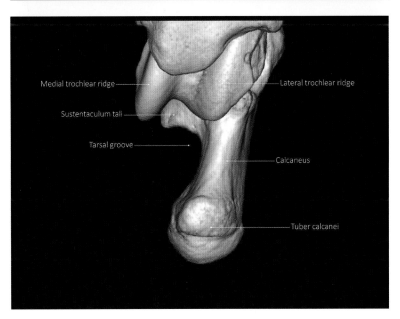

Figure 11.24 3D representation of the flexed DPI projection of the tarsus.

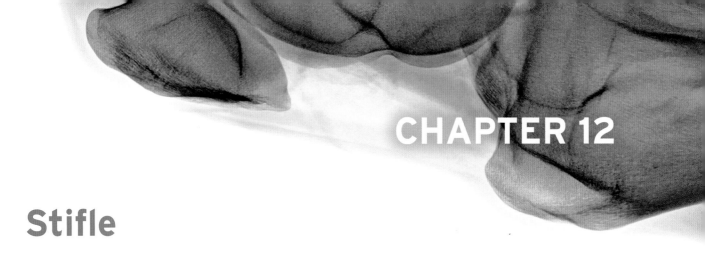

CHAPTER 12

Stifle

Indications

Stifle radiography in the performance horse is a fairly routine procedure in equine practice.

Indications for performing radiographs of the stifle include:

- Lameness localized to the stifle by diagnostic analgesia (femoropatellar joint block, lateral femorotibial joint block or medial femorotibial joint block)
- Soft tissue swelling, including joint effusion
- Signs of trauma, such as wounds
- Abnormal position of the patella
- As part of a pre-purchase or pre-sales examination.

Equipment

For a complete study of the stifle the following equipment is required:

- Portable X-ray machine may be sufficient, depending on the size and condition of the horse. Caudocranial projections may require higher exposures and the use of a high-output X-ray machine may be necessary

- Large plates (35 × 43 cm) are recommended
- Plate holder: a short-handled plate holder may be used depending on the horse
- Radiation safety equipment: lead gowns, lead gloves and thyroid protectors.

Preparation

If necessary, brush or wash the area to reduce artefacts caused by dirt. Sedation of the patient is advised.

Radiographic protocol

A standard radiographic examination of the stifle usually includes at least two radiographs:

- Lateromedial (LM)
- Caudocranial (CdCr).

Additional projections:

- Caudo 60° lateral-craniomedial oblique (Cd60L-CrMO)
- Flexed lateromedial (flexed LM)
- Cranioproximal-craniodistal oblique (CrPr-CrDiO) or 'skyline' view of the patella.

Lateromedial (LM) (Figs 12.1–12.4)

1. Stand the horse square with the cannon bone vertical to the ground in each direction and ensure that all limbs are equally weight-bearing. The limb to be examined should be positioned caudal to the contralateral limb and fully weight-bearing; this may facilitate plate positioning.
2. Place the plate in portrait orientation on the medial side of the stifle as close as possible to the limb. It is often tricky to extend the plate far enough up in the groin region; angling the plate alongside the abdomen of the horse is recommended.
3. Place a R/L marker on the dorsal side of the plate.
4. Position the X-ray machine on the lateral side of the stifle.
5. Focus–film distance: 100 cm.
6. Use a horizontal X-ray beam perpendicularly aligned to the limb and plate.
7. Centre the X-ray beam at the level of the femorotibial joint (proximal to the tibial crest), about 10 cm caudal to the cranial edge of the leg.
8. Collimate tightly around the stifle to reduce scatter.
9. Exposure guide: 75 kVp, 30 mAs.

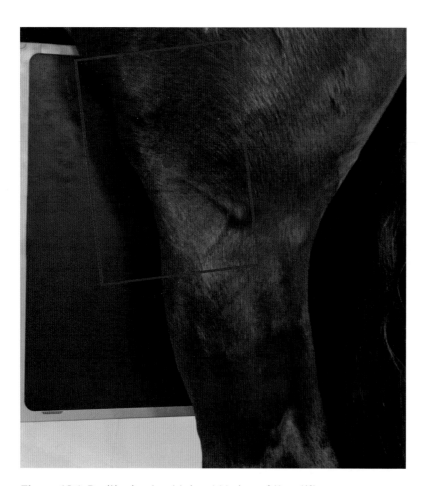

Figure 12.1 Positioning to obtain a LM view of the stifle.

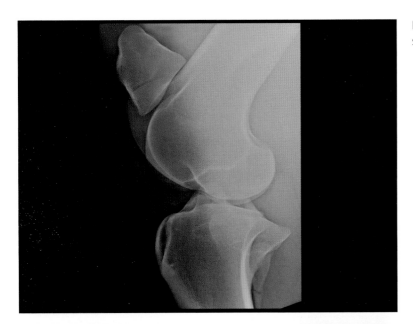

Figure 12.2 LM projection of the stifle.

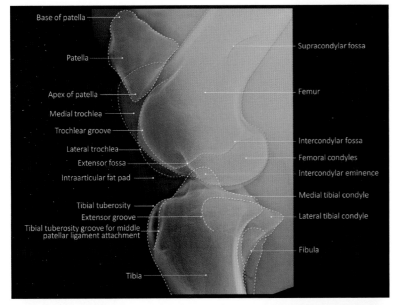

Figure 12.3 Radiographic anatomy of the LM projection of the stifle.

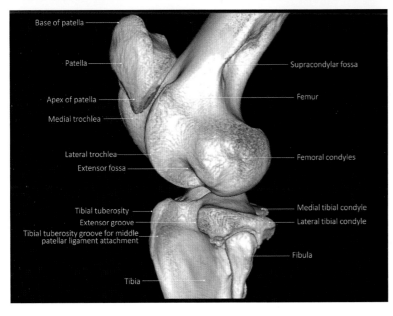

Figure 12.4 3D representation of the LM projection of the stifle.

Caudocranial (CdCr) (Figs 12.5–12.8)

1. Stand the horse square with the cannon bone vertical to the ground in each direction and ensure that all limbs are equally weight-bearing. The limb to be examined should be positioned caudal to the contralateral limb and be fully weight-bearing; this may facilitate plate positioning.
2. Place the plate in portrait orientation cranial to the stifle as close as possible to the limb.
3. Place a R/L marker on the lateral side of the plate.
4. Position the X-ray machine caudal to the stifle.
5. Focus–film distance: 100 cm.
6. Angle the X-ray beam downward along the tibial plateau, approximately 10–20 degrees to the horizontal. It may be helpful to palpate the tibial plateau and mark it with some tape.
7. Centre the X-ray beam at the level of the tibial plateau.
8. Collimate tightly around the stifle to reduce scatter.
9. Exposure guide: 90 kVp, 30 mAs.

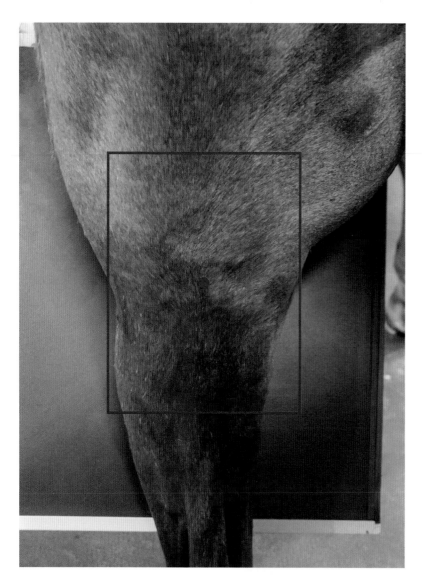

Figure 12.5 Positioning to obtain a CdCr view of the stifle.

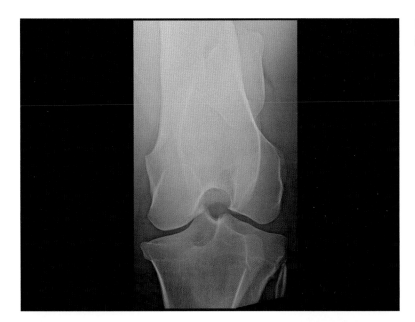

Figure 12.6 CdCr projection of the stifle.

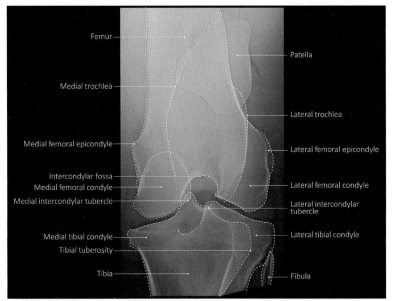

Figure 12.7 Radiographic anatomy of the CdCr projection of the stifle.

Femur

Medial trochlea

Medial femoral epicondyle

Intercondylar fossa
Medial femoral condyle
Medial intercondylar tubercle

Medial tibial condyle
Tibial tuberosity

Tibia

Patella

Lateral trochlea

Lateral femoral epicondyle

Lateral femoral condyle

Lateral intercondylar tubercle

Lateral tibial condyle

Fibula

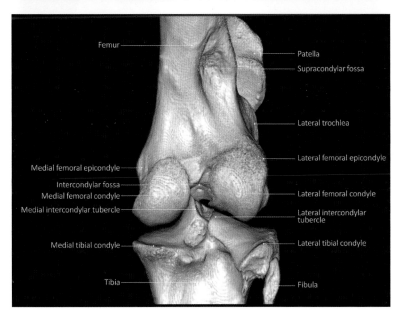

Figure 12.8 3D representation of the CdCr projection of the stifle.

Femur

Medial femoral epicondyle

Intercondylar fossa
Medial femoral condyle
Medial intercondylar tubercle

Medial tibial condyle

Tibia

Patella
Supracondylar fossa

Lateral trochlea

Lateral femoral epicondyle

Lateral femoral condyle

Lateral intercondylar tubercle

Lateral tibial condyle

Fibula

Caudo 60° lateral-craniomedial oblique (Cd60L-CrMO) (Figs 12.9-12.12)

1. Stand the horse square with the cannon bone vertical to the ground in each direction and ensure that all limbs are equally weight-bearing.
2. Place the plate in portrait orientation craniomedially to the joint as close as possible to the limb.
3. Place a R/L marker on the lateral side of the plate.
4. Position the X-ray machine caudolaterally to the limb at a 60-degree angle from the sagittal plane of the limb.
5. Focus–film distance: 100 cm.
6. Angle the X-ray beam downward along the tibial plateau, approximately 10–20 degrees to the horizontal.
7. Centre the X-ray beam at the level of the femorotibial joint (proximal to the tibial crest), about 10 cm caudal to the cranial edge of the leg.
8. Collimate tightly around the stifle to reduce scatter.
9. Exposure guide: 75 kVp, 30 mAs.

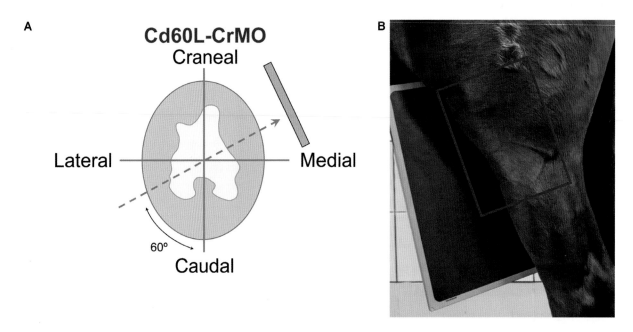

Figure 12.9 Diagram showing how to obtain a Cd60L-CrMO view of the stifle (A) and positioning to obtain the same view (B).

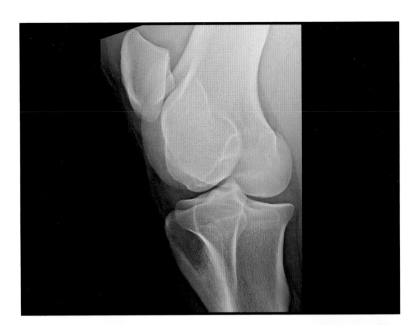

Figure 12.10 Cd60L-CrMO projection of the stifle.

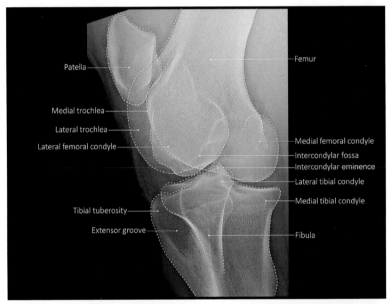

Figure 12.11 Radiographic anatomy of the Cd60L-CrMO projection of the stifle.

Patella

Medial trochlea

Lateral trochlea

Lateral femoral condyle

Tibial tuberosity

Extensor groove

Femur

Medial femoral condyle

Intercondylar fossa

Intercondylar eminence

Lateral tibial condyle

Medial tibial condyle

Fibula

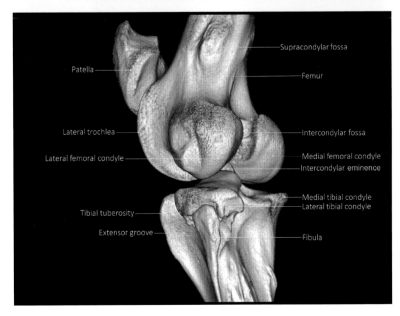

Figure 12.12 3D representation of the Cd60L-CrMO projection of the stifle.

Patella

Lateral trochlea

Lateral femoral condyle

Tibial tuberosity

Extensor groove

Supracondylar fossa

Femur

Intercondylar fossa

Medial femoral condyle

Intercondylar eminence

Medial tibial condyle

Lateral tibial condyle

Fibula

Flexed lateromedial (flexed LM) (Figs 12.13–12.16)

1. Flex the stifle with gloved hands by retracting the limb so that the tibia is approximately horizontal to the ground.
2. Place the plate in landscape orientation on the medial side of the stifle as close as possible to the limb and as high up as possible in the groin region.
3. Place a R/L marker on the dorsal side of the plate.
4. Position the X-ray machine on the lateral side of the limb.
5. Focus–film distance: 100 cm.
6. Use a horizontal X-ray beam perpendicularly aligned to the limb and plate.
7. Centre the X-ray beam at the level of the femorotibial joint (proximal to the tibial crest), about 10 cm caudal to the cranial edge of the leg.
8. Collimate tightly around the stifle to reduce scatter.
9. Exposure guide: 75 kVp, 30 mAs.

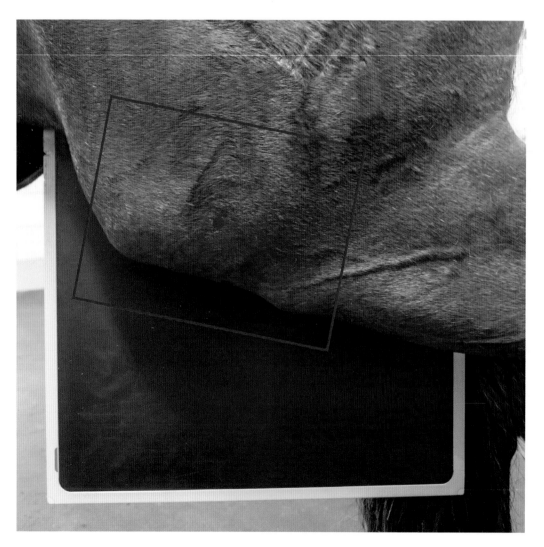

Figure 12.13 Positioning to obtain a flexed LM view of the stifle.

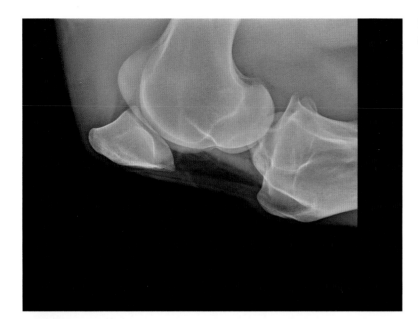

Figure 12.14 Flexed LM projection of the stifle.

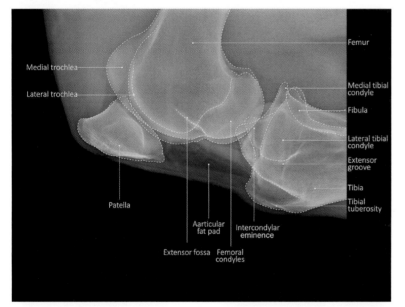

Figure 12.15 Radiographic anatomy of the flexed LM projection of the stifle.

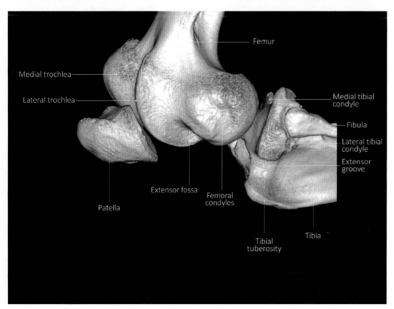

Figure 12.16 3D representation of the flexed LM projection of the stifle.

Cranioproximal-craniodistal oblique (CrPr-CrDiO) or 'skyline' view of the patella (Figs 12.17–12.20)

1. Flex the stifle with gloved hands by retracting the limb so that the tibia is approximately horizontal to the ground. Adducting the flexed limb may facilitate positioning by rotating the stifle outwards.
2. Place the plate in a horizontal position facing upwards underneath the patella.
3. Place a R/L marker on the lateral side of the plate.
4. Position the X-ray machine above the stifle. A 100 cm focus–film distance is usually not possible since the X-ray machine cannot be positioned high enough in relation to the patella.
5. Angle the X-ray beam downward.
6. Centre the X-ray beam on the patella.
7. Collimate tightly to reduce scatter.
8. Exposure guide: 70 kVp, 10 mAs.

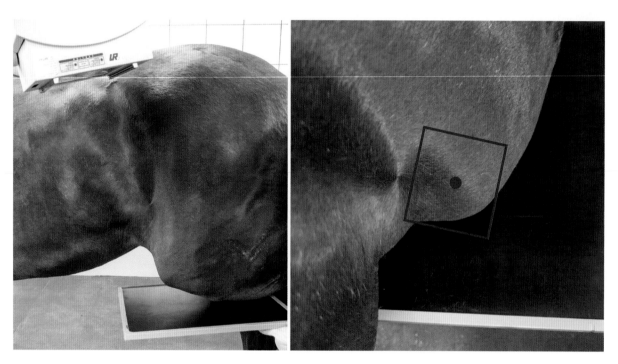

Figure 12.17 Positioning to obtain a CrPr-CrDiO view of the stifle.

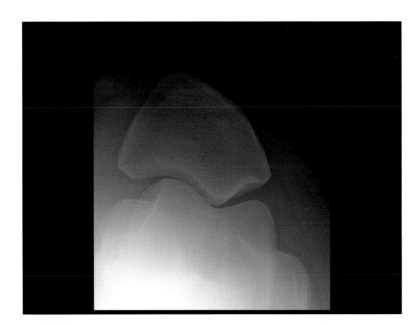

Figure 12.18 CrPr-CrDiO projection of the stifle.

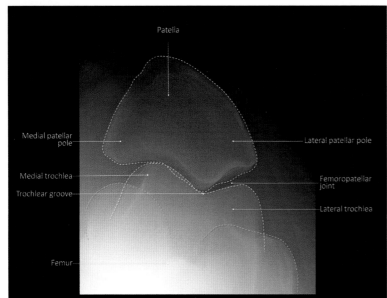

Figure 12.19 Radiographic anatomy of the CrPr-CrDiO projection of the stifle.

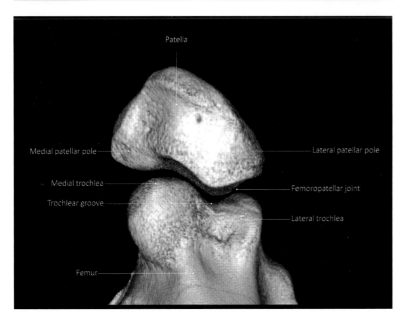

Figure 12.20 3D representation of the CrPr-CrDiO projection of the stifle.

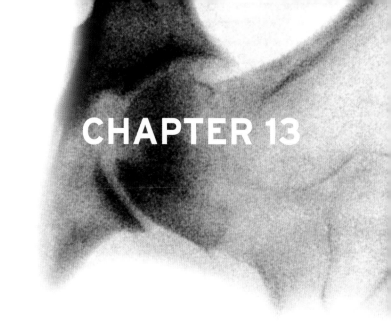

CHAPTER 13

Pelvis

Indications

Radiography of the pelvis is not a commonly performed procedure in horses mainly because pelvis-associated lameness is uncommon, but pelvic radiographs may be useful in diagnosing fractures, coxofemoral (sub)luxations or osteoarthritis.

Indications for performing radiographs of the pelvis include:

- Hind limb lameness that cannot be localized by diagnostic analgesia to other areas of the limb
- External asymmetry or muscle atrophy of the pelvic region
- Positive rectal examination: crepitus or asymmetry
- Scintigraphic or ultrasonographic findings suggestive of pelvic disease.

Equipment

For a complete study of the pelvis the following equipment is required:

- High-output X-ray generator
- Large plates (35 × 43 cm)
- Grids are helpful to reduce scatter and hence improve image quality. For example, the use of two focused grids with grid lines at right angles to each other and a sheet of lead placed behind the plate is recommended for VD projections

- Standing projections: ceiling/wall-mounted bucky and plate holder is highly recommended. Handholding of the plate must be avoided due to the high exposures and the scatter radiation involved
- Recumbent projections: general anaesthesia equipment and a tunnel block to allow positioning of the plates under the horse
- Radiation safety equipment: lead gowns and thyroid protectors.

Preparation

Sedation of the patient is advised for standing projections. Rectum emptying is useful to reduce artefacts created by overlying faecal material. General anaesthesia is paramount for recumbent projections.

Radiographic protocol

Radiographic protocol of the pelvis depends on the suspected disease. Several different projections have been described:

- Ventrodorsal under general anaesthesia (GA VD)
- Cranioventral-caudodorsal oblique (CrV-CdDO) in the standing horse
- Right 30° dorsal-left ventral oblique (R30D-LVO) and Left 30° dorsal-right ventral oblique (L30D-RVO) for the coxofemoral joint.

Ventrodorsal under general anaesthesia (VD GA) (Figs 13.1–13.4)

1. Position the horse in dorsal recumbency in a frog-leg position.
2. Place the plate facing upwards in a tunnel block under the horse's pelvis.
3. Indicate right/left with a marker.
4. Position the X-ray machine dorsal to the pelvis.
5. Focus–film distance: 120 cm. Adjust the focus–film distance to the distance specified for the grid.
6. Use a vertical X-ray beam.
7. X-ray beam centring depends on the area of interest, as several overlapping views are required for a comprehensive radiographic examination of the pelvis. In a standard adult horse, seven separate views are described:

   – Midline views; centred on the respective anatomical landmarks:

     ○ Tubera ischii
     ○ Coxofemoral joints and obturadora foramina
     ○ Sacroiliac and lumbosacral joints.

   – Tuber coxae
   – Coxofemoral joints: the limb to be radiographed is tilted nearer to the plate by slightly rolling the horse.

8. Exposure guide: 150 kVp, 250 mAs.

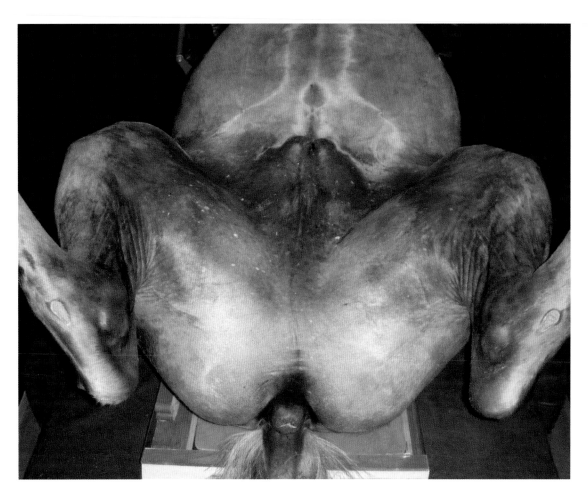

Figure 13.1 Positioning to obtain a VD view of the pelvis under general anaesthesia.

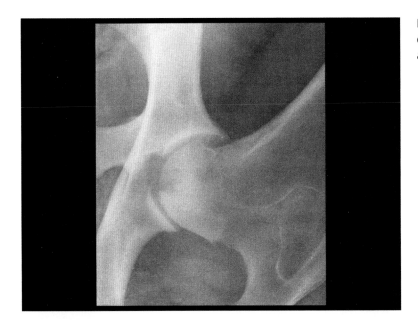

Figure 13.2 VD projection of the coxofemoral joint under general anaesthesia.

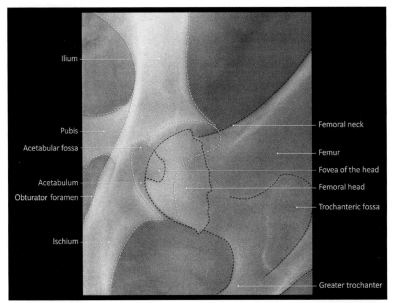

Figure 13.3 Radiographic anatomy of the VD projection of the coxofemoral joint under general anaesthesia.

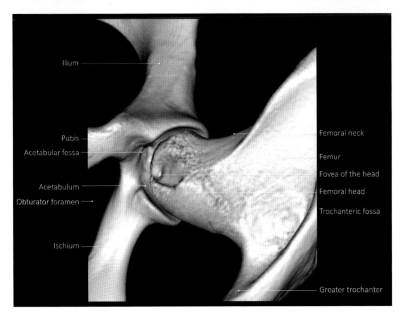

Figure 13.4 3D representation of the VD projection of the coxofemoral joint under general anaesthesia.

Cranioventral-caudodorsal oblique (CrV-CdDO) in the standing horse (Figs 13.5–13.8)

1. Stand the horse square with the hind limbs abducted as far as possible and ensure all limbs are equally weight-bearing.
2. Place the plate in landscape orientation dorsal to the pelvic region, following the inclination of the pelvis.
3. Indicate right/left with a marker.
4. Position the X-ray machine ventral to the horse's abdomen in front of the hind limbs.
5. Focus–film distance: 120 cm. Adjust the focus–film distance to the distance specified for the grid.
6. Angle the X-ray beam upward 10–25 degrees from the vertical.
7. X-ray beam centring depends on the area of interest as several overlapping views are required for a comprehensive radiographic examination of the pelvis.
8. Collimate tightly around the area of interest to reduce scatter.
9. Exposure guide: 150 kVp, 200 mAs.

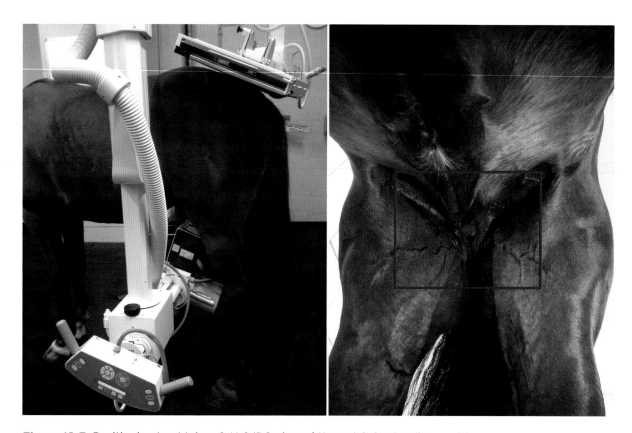

Figure 13.5 Positioning to obtain a CrV-CdDO view of the pelvis in standing position.

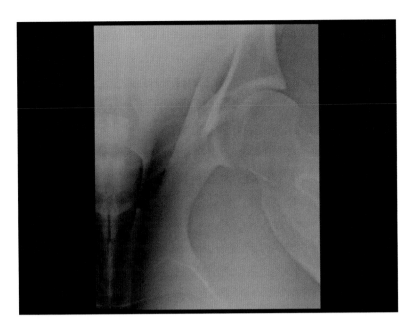

Figure 13.6 CrV-CdDO projection of the pelvis in standing position.

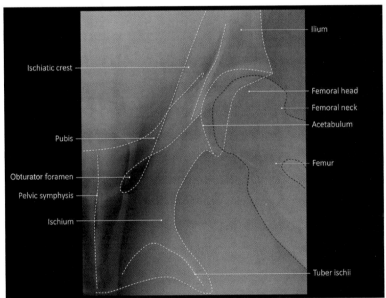

Figure 13.7 Radiographic anatomy of the CrV-CdDO projection of the pelvis in standing position.

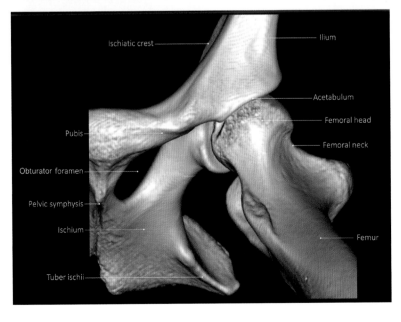

Figure 13.8 3D representation of the CrV-CdDO projection of the pelvis in standing position.

Right 30° dorsal-left ventral oblique (R30D-LVO) and Left 30° dorsal-right ventral oblique (L30D-RVO) for the coxofemoral joint (Figs 13.9–13.12)

1. Stand the horse square with all limbs equally weight-bearing.
2. Place the plate vertically in landscape orientation on the side of the leg of interest and position the X-ray machine on the contralateral side above the pelvis.

   – R30D-LVO: highlights the left coxofemoral joint.
   – L30D-RVO: highlights the right coxofemoral joint.

3. Indicate right/left (plate's side) with a marker.
4. Focus–film distance: 120 cm. Adjust the focus–film distance to the distance specified for the grid.
5. Angle the X-ray beam downward 30 degrees to the horizontal.
6. Centre the X-ray beam between the greater trochanter on the affected side and the base of the tail; an alternative method would be to centre on a spot that corresponds to two thirds of the distance between the tuber sacrale and tuber ischii on the side of the X-ray machine.
7. Collimate around the area of interest.
8. Exposure guide: 110 kVp, 140 mAs.

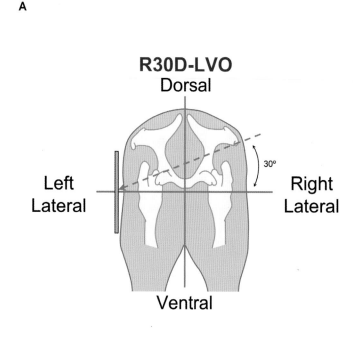

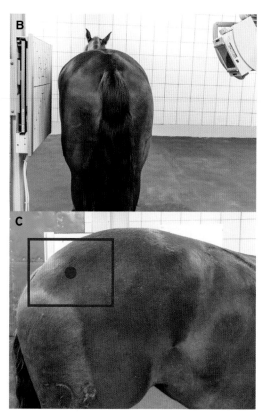

Figure 13.9 Diagram showing how to obtain the R30D-LVO view for the left coxofemoral joint (A) and positioning to obtain the same view (B and C).

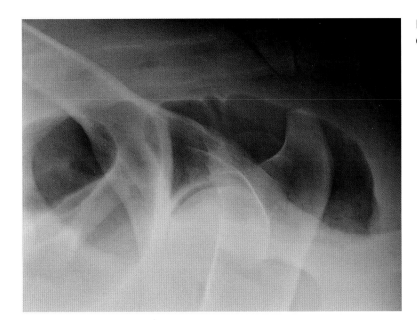

Figure 13.10 R30D-LVO projection of the left coxofemoral joint.

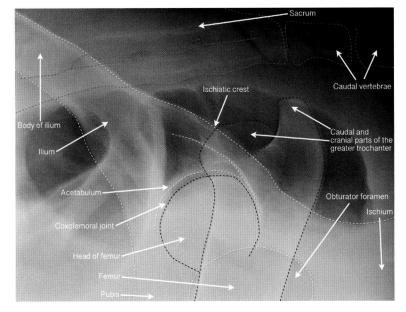

Figure 13.11 Radiographic anatomy of the R30D-LVO projection of the left coxofemoral joint.

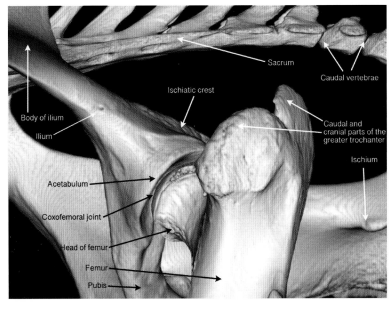

Figure 13.12 3D representation of the R30D-LVO projection of the left coxofemoral joint.

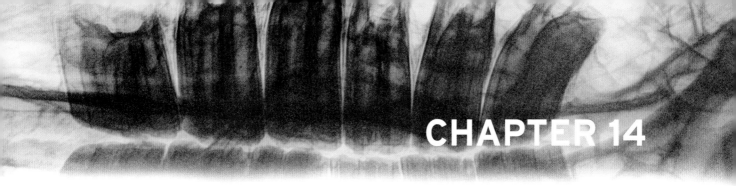

CHAPTER 14

Head

Indications

The head is one of the most anatomically complex regions of the body and a wide range of disorders affecting the different structures can be found.

Indications for performing radiographs of the head include:

- Nasal discharge
- Soft tissue or osseous swellings
- Clinical signs associated with dental disease (quidding, weight loss, discharging tracts, malodorous breath, etc.)
- Lacerations or wounds
- Less specific clinical indications include: poor performance, equitation issues, headshaking.

Equipment

For a complete study of the head, the following equipment is required:

- Portable X-ray machine is sufficient
- Large plates (35 × 43 cm)
- Rope/webbing headcollar to avoid metal artefacts
- Plate holder is highly recommended (ceiling/wall-mounted or handheld)
- Head stand
- Mouth gag
- Radiation safety equipment: lead gowns, lead gloves and thyroid protectors.

Preparation

If necessary, brush or wash the area to reduce artefacts caused by dirt. Put on a rope headcollar. Sedation of the patient is recommended.

Radiographic protocol

Several projections have been described for assessing the different parts of this region, the most common views being the laterolateral and dorsoventral. However, additional specific views have been described for more specific areas (Table 14.1).

Table 14.1 Radiographic projections for evaluation of the equine head.

Examination area	Radiographic projection	Structures evaluated
Premaxilla (incisor bone) and rostral mandible	*Laterolateral (LL)*	Incisive bone and rostral mandible
	Dorsoventral (DV)	Incisive bone and rostral mandible
	Intraoral dorsoventral (DV)	Maxillary incisors and incisive bone
	Intraoral ventrodorsal (VD)	Mandibular incisors and rostral mandible
Nasal cavity and paranasal sinuses	*Laterolateral (LL)*	Nasal cavity and paranasal sinuses
	Dorsoventral (DV)	Nasal cavity, paranasal sinuses and zygomatic arch
	Right 30° dorsal-left ventral oblique (R30D-LVO) and Left 30° dorsal-right ventral oblique (L30D-RVO)	Maxillary cheek teeth, paranasal sinuses and orbit
	Right 75° dorsal-left ventral oblique (R75D-LVO) and Left 75° dorsal-right ventral oblique (L75D-RVO)	Maxillary sinuses and orbit
	Open-mouth Right 15° ventral-left dorsal oblique (R15V-LDO) and Left 15° ventral-right dorsal oblique (L15V-RDO)	Maxillary cheek teeth erupted crowns
	Offset mandible dorsoventral (DV)	Maxillary cheek teeth
Mandible (body)	*Laterolateral (LL)*	Mandible (body)
	Right 45° ventral-left dorsal oblique (R45V-LDO) and Left 45° ventral-right dorsal oblique (L45V-RDO)	Mandible (body) and mandibular cheek teeth
	Open-mouth Right 10° dorsal-left ventral oblique (R10D-LVO) and Left 10° dorsal-right ventral oblique (L10D-RVO)	Mandibular cheek teeth erupted crowns
Caudal skull	*Laterolateral (LL)*	Cranial vault, temporomandibular joint, tympanohyoid articulation and vertical mandibular rami
	Ventrodorsal (VD)	Cranial vault, petrous temporal bone, stylohyoid bone, vertical mandibular rami, paracondylar processes, occipital condyles and zygomatic arch
	Rostro 35° latero 50° ventral-caudodorsal oblique (R35L50V-CdDO)	Temporomandibular joint
Pharynx	*Laterolateral (LL)*	Pharynx, larynx, guttural pouches and soft palate

Laterolateral (LL) (Figs 14.1–14.9)

1. Position the head with the nose vertical with the help of a head stand (or bale of shavings, etc., if no headstand available). Avoid any tilting or rotation of the head. Extension of the head and neck may facilitate the evaluation of the pharyngeal and laryngeal region.
2. Place the plate on the affected side in a vertical position and align with the area of interest.
3. Indicate right/left (plate's side) with a marker.
4. Position the X-ray machine on the other side of the head.
5. Focus–film distance: 100 cm.
6. Use a horizontal X-ray beam, perpendicular to the long axis of the head and plate.
7. X-ray beam centring depends on the area of interest:

   - Rostral head: corner of the mouth (Fig. 14.1)
   - Paranasal sinuses: dorsal to the rostral third of the facial crest (Fig. 14.2)
   - Caudal head: middle third of the caudal border of the mandibular ramus (Fig. 14.3).

8. Align the field of view with the long axis of the nose for the rostral head and paranasal sinuses and collimate around the area of interest.
9. Exposure guide:

   - Rostral head and paranasal sinuses: 60 kVp, 15 mAs
   - Caudal head: 70 kVp, 40 mAs.

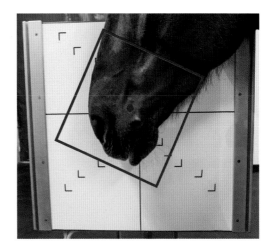

Figure 14.1 Positioning to obtain a LL view of the rostral aspect of the head.

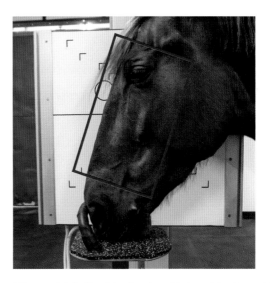

Figure 14.2 Positioning to obtain a LL view of the head at the level of the paranasal sinuses.

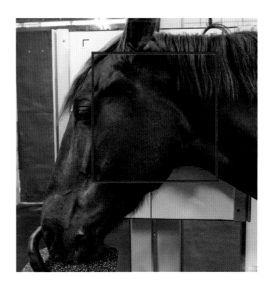

Figure 14.3 Positioning to obtain a LL view of the caudal aspect of the head.

Figure 14.4
LL projection of the rostral aspect of the head.

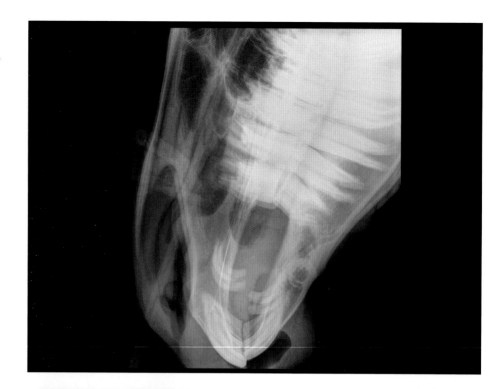

Figure 14.5
Radiographic anatomy of the LL projection of the rostral aspect of the head.

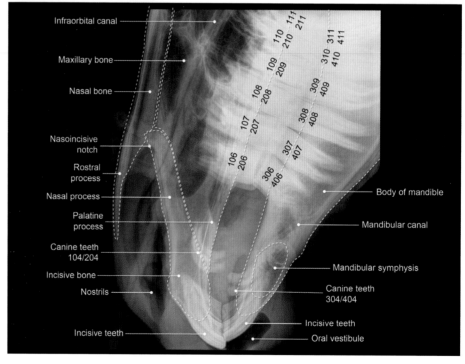

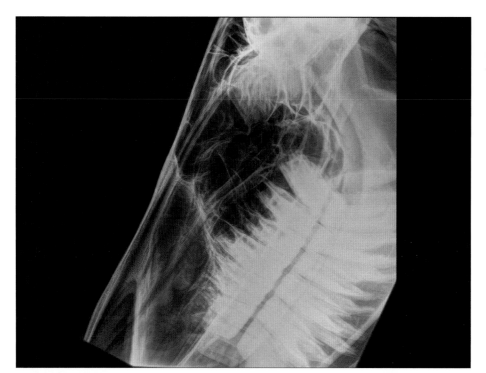

Figure 14.6
LL projection of the head at the level of the paranasal sinuses.

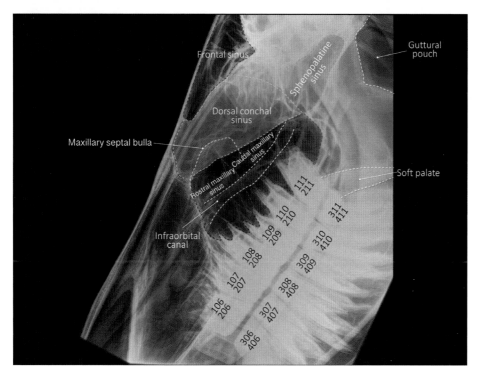

Figure 14.7
Radiographic anatomy of the LL projection of the head at the level of the paranasal sinuses.

Figure 14.8 LL projection of the caudal aspect of the head.

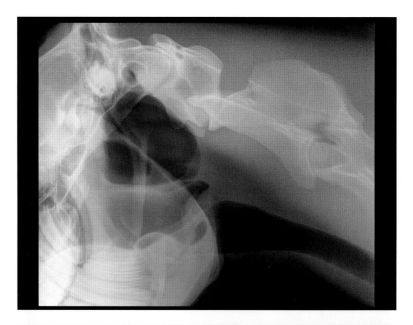

Figure 14.9 Radiographic anatomy of the LL projection of the caudal aspect of the head.

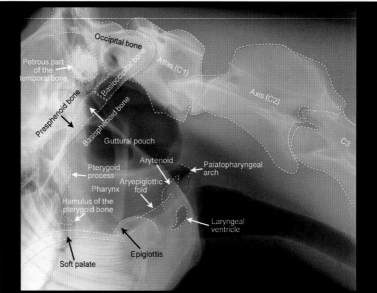

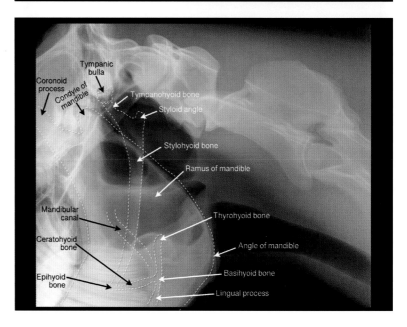

Dorsoventral (DV) (Figs 14.10–14.15)

1. Position the head with the nose extended rostrally. Care must be taken to avoid any rotation/tilting of the head. A head stand may facilitate the positioning when evaluating the paranasal sinuses.
2. Place the plate ventral to the head, along the mandible.
3. Indicate right/left with a marker.
4. Position the X-ray machine dorsal to the head.
5. Focus–film distance: 100 cm.
6. Orientate the X-ray beam perpendicular to the plate.
7. Centre the X-ray beam in the midline of the head. Centring depends on the area of interest:

   – Rostral head: in the midline of the head at the level of the corner of the mouth (Fig. 14.10).
   – Paranasal sinuses: in the midline of the head at the level of the rostral third of the facial crest (Fig. 14.11).

8. Collimate around the head.
9. Exposure guide:

   – Rostral head: 60 kVp, 25 mAs
   – Paranasal sinuses: 75 kVp, 30 mAs.

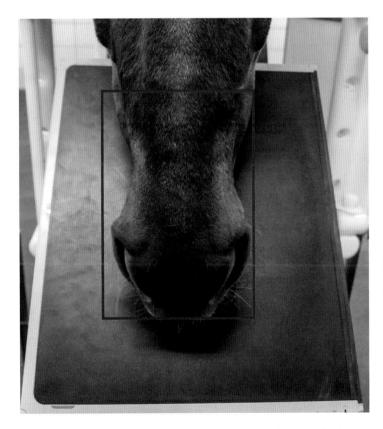

Figure 14.10 Positioning to obtain a DV view of the rostral aspect of the head.

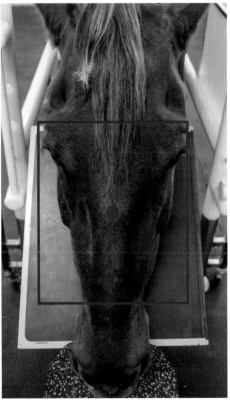

Figure 14.11 Positioning to obtain a DV view of the head at the level of the paranasal sinuses.

Figure 14.12
DV projection of the rostral aspect of the head.

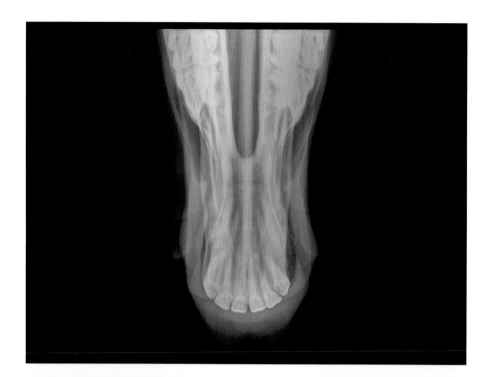

Figure 14.13
Radiographic anatomy of the DV projection of the rostral aspect of the head.

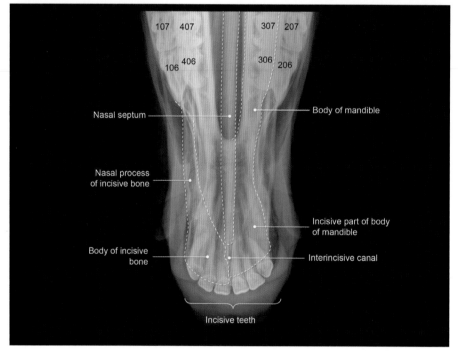

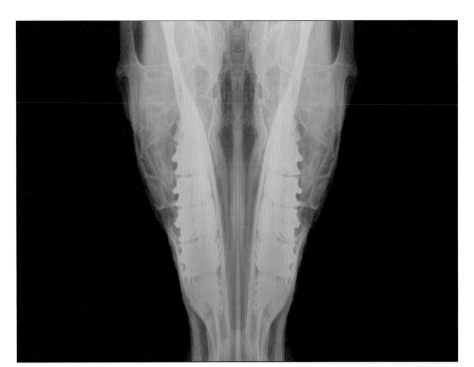

Figure 14.14
DV projection of the head at the level of the paranasal sinuses.

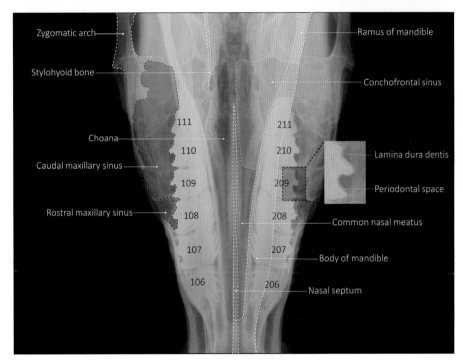

Zygomatic arch

Stylohyoid bone

Choana

Caudal maxillary sinus

Rostral maxillary sinus

Ramus of mandible

Conchofrontal sinus

111
110
109
108
107
106

211
210
209
208
207
206

Lamina dura dentis

Periodontal space

Common nasal meatus

Body of mandible

Nasal septum

Figure 14.15
Radiographic anatomy of the DV projection of the head at the level of the paranasal sinuses.

Ventrodorsal (VD) (Figs 14.16–14.18)

1. Position the head with the nose extended rostrally as much as possible with the help of a head stand. Avoid any tilting or rotation of the head.
2. Place the plate dorsal to the head aligned with the nose/frontal region.
3. Indicate right/left with a marker.
4. Position the X-ray machine ventral to the head.
5. Focus–film distance: 100 cm.
6. Orientate the X-ray beam perpendicular to the plate.
7. Centre the X-ray beam in the midline of the head at the level of the temporomandibular joint.
8. Collimate around the head.
9. Exposure guide: 90 kVp, 55 mAs.

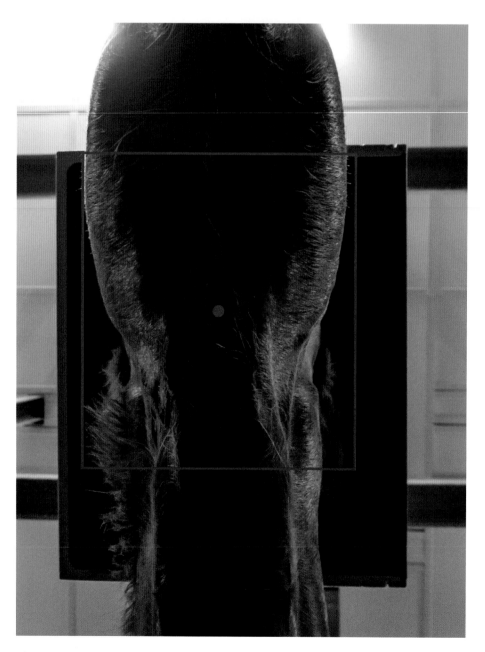

Figure 14.16 Positioning to obtain a VD view of the caudal aspect of the head.

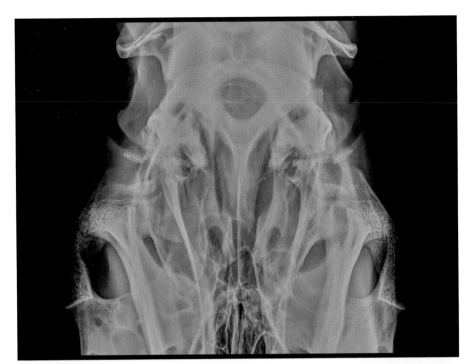

Figure 14.17
VD projection of the
caudal aspect of
the head.

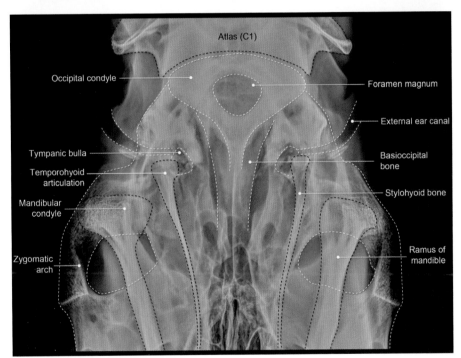

Figure 14.18
Radiographic anatomy
of the VD projection of
the caudal aspect of the
head.

Intraoral dorsoventral (DV) for maxillary incisors (Figs 14.19-14.21)

1. Keep the mouth open with a gag that leaves the incisive region free or use a radiolucent gag.
2. Place the plate facing upwards in the mouth between the incisors, as far caudally as possible.
3. Indicate right/left with a marker.
4. Position the X-ray machine dorsal to the head.
5. Focus–film distance: 100 cm.
6. Orientate the X-ray beam obliquely downwards, directed 90 degrees to the plane that bisects the angle between the incisor reserve crown-root and the plate.
7. Centre the X-ray beam in the midline of the head on the central incisors.
8. Collimate around the area of interest.
9. Exposure guide: 50 kVp, 10 mAs.

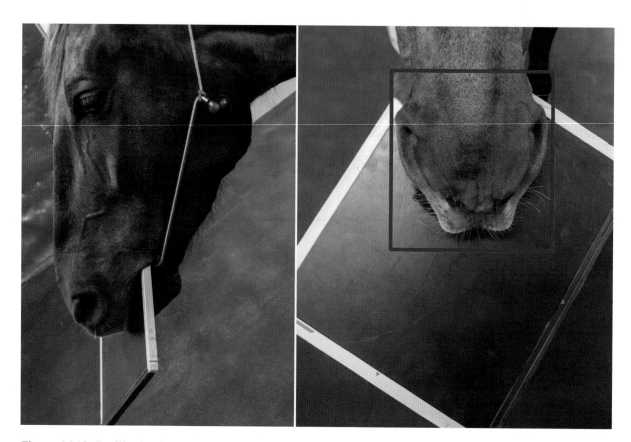

Figure 14.19 Positioning to obtain an intraoral DV view of the premaxilla.

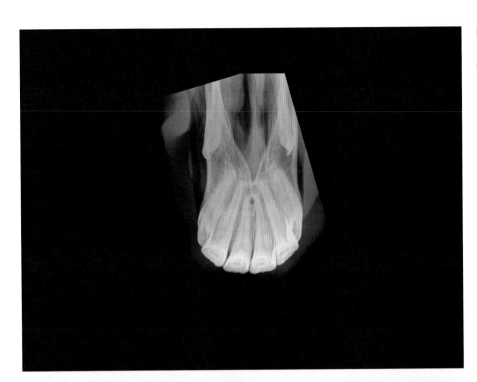

Figure 14.20
Intraoral DV projection
of the premaxilla.

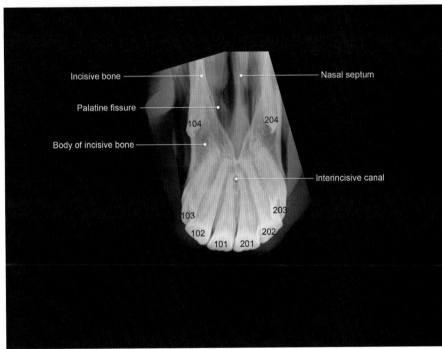

Figure 14.21
Radiographic anatomy
of the intraoral DV
projection of the
premaxilla.

Intraoral ventrodorsal (VD) for mandibular incisors (Figs 14.22–14.24)

1. Keep the mouth open with a gag that leaves the incisive region free or use a radiolucent gag.
2. Place the plate facing downwards in the mouth between the incisors, as far caudally as possible.
3. Indicate right/left with a marker.
4. Position the X-ray machine ventral to the head.
5. Focus–film distance: 100 cm.
6. Orientate the X-ray beam obliquely upwards, directed 90 degrees to the plane that bisects the angle between the incisor reserve crown-root and the plate.
7. Centre the X-ray beam in the midline of the head on the central incisors.
8. Collimate around the area of interest.
9. Exposure guide: 50 kVp, 10 mAs.

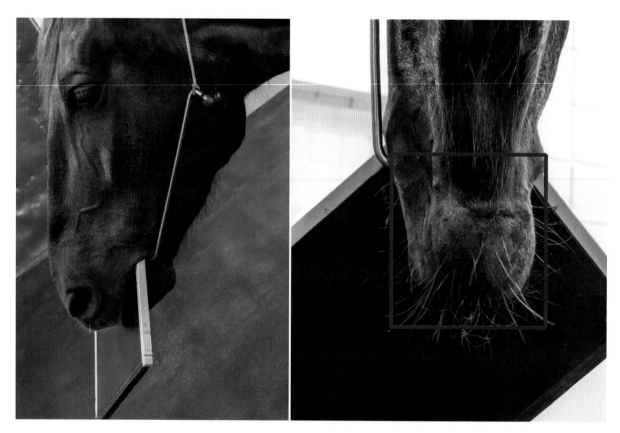

Figure 14.22 Positioning to obtain an intraoral VD view of the rostral aspect of the mandible.

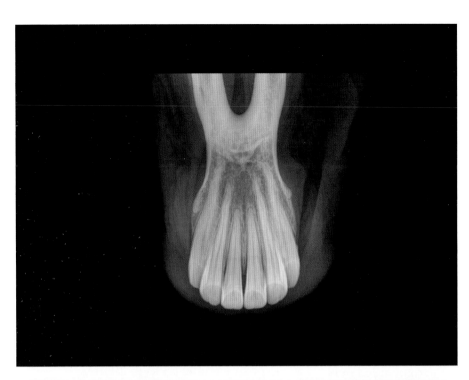

Figure 14.23
Intraoral VD projection
of the rostral aspect of
the mandible.

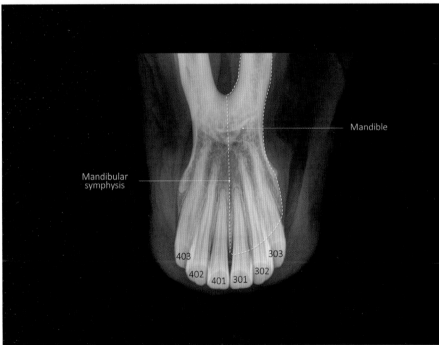

Figure 14.24
Radiographic anatomy
of the intraoral VD
projection of the rostral
aspect of the mandible.

Right 30° dorsal-left ventral oblique (R30D-LVO) and Left 30° dorsal-right ventral oblique (L30D-RVO) for maxillary cheek teeth (Figs 14.25–14.27)

1. Position the head straight (avoid tilting or rotation) with the nose vertical with the help of a head stand. Alternatively, the head can be stretched out so that the nose is horizontal. Both ways standardize head position and help to angle the beam correctly.

2. Place the plate on the affected side in a vertical position and aligned with the area of interest.

   – R30D-LVO: outlines the left-sided maxillary cheek teeth and paranasal sinuses.
   – L30D-RVO: outlines the right-sided maxillary cheek teeth and paranasal sinuses.

3. Indicate right/left (plate's side) with a marker.

4. Position the X-ray machine on the other side of the head.

5. Focus–film distance: 100 cm.

6. Angle the X-ray beam, so that the X-ray beam hits the dorsal plane (hard palate) at a 30-degree downward angle. Alternatively, the X-ray beam can be angled downwards 75 degrees when evaluation of the paranasal sinuses is required.

7. Centre the X-ray beam dorsal to the rostral third of the facial crest.

8. Align the field of view with the long axis of the nose by tilting the X-ray machine if necessary and collimate around the area of interest.

9. Exposure guide: 65 kVp, 20 mAs.

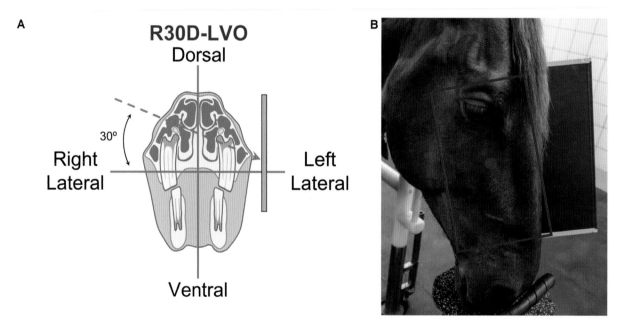

Figure 14.25 Diagram (A) and positioning (B) to obtain an R30D-LVO view of the head that outlines the left-sided maxillary cheek teeth and paranasal sinuses.

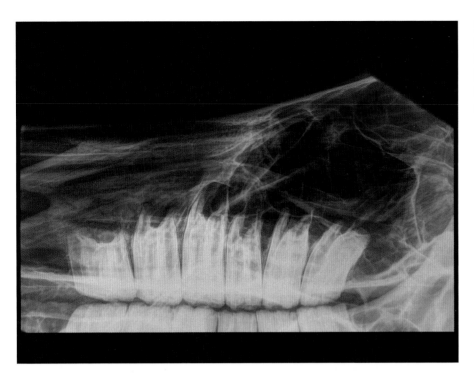

Figure 14.26
R30D-LVO projection of the head that outlines the left-sided maxillary cheek teeth and paranasal sinuses.

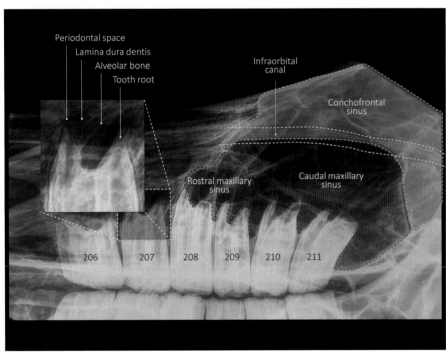

Figure 14.27
Radiographic anatomy of the R30D-LVO projection of the head that outlines the left-sided maxillary cheek teeth and paranasal sinuses.

Right 45⁰ ventral-left dorsal oblique (R45V-LDO) and Left 45⁰ ventral-right dorsal oblique (L45V-RDO) for mandibular cheek teeth (Figs 14.28–14.30)

1. Position the head straight (avoid tilting or rotation) with the nose vertical with the help of a head stand. Alternatively, the head can be stretched out so that the nose is horizontal. Both ways standardize head position and help to angle the beam correctly.
2. Place the plate on the affected side in a vertical position and aligned with the area of interest.

   – R45V-LDO: outlines the left-sided mandibular cheek teeth.
   – L45V-RDO: outlines the right-sided mandibular cheek teeth.

3. Indicate right/left (plate's side) with a marker.
4. Position the X-ray machine on the other side of the head.
5. Focus–film distance: 100 cm.
6. Angle the X-ray beam, so that the X-ray beam hits the dorsal plane (hard palate) at a 45-degree upward angle.
7. Centre the X-ray beam in the middle of the body of the affected mandible.
8. Align the field of view with the long axis of the mandible and collimate around the area of interest.
9. Exposure guide: 80 kVp, 20 mAs.

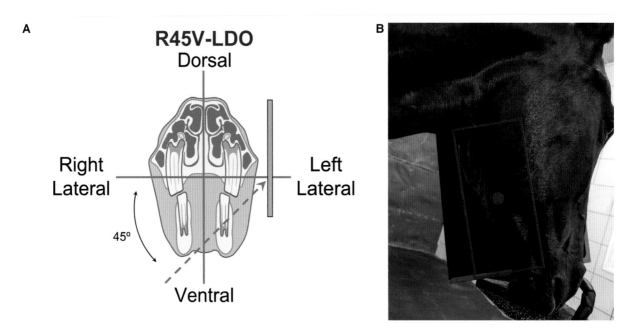

Figure 14.28 Diagram (A) and positioning (B) to obtain an R45V-LDO view of the head that outlines the left-sided mandibular cheek teeth.

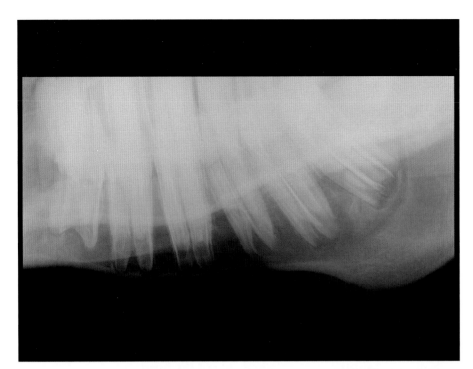

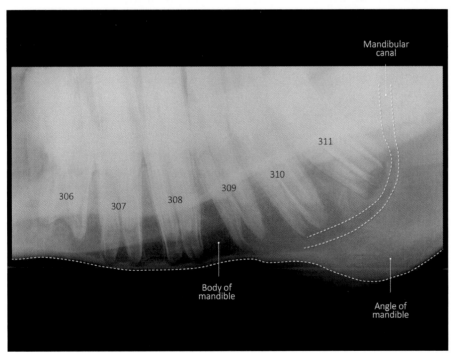

Figure 14.30
Radiographic anatomy
of the R45V-LDO
projection of the head
that outlines the
left-sided mandibular
cheek teeth.

Right 15° ventral-left dorsal oblique (R15V-LDO) and Left 15° ventral-right dorsal oblique (L15V-RDO) (Figs 14.31 and 14.32)

1. Keep the mouth open with a gag that leaves the cheek teeth free.
2. Place the plate on the affected side in a vertical position and aligned with the area of interest.

   – R15V-LDO: outlines the left-sided maxillary cheek teeth erupted crown.
   – L15V-RDO: outlines the right-sided maxillary cheek teeth erupted crown.

3. Indicate right/left (plate's side) with a marker.
4. Position the X-ray machine on the other side of the head.
5. Focus–film distance: 100 cm.
6. Angle the X-ray beam, so that the X-ray beam hits the dorsal plane (hard palate) at a 15-degree upward angle.
7. Centre the X-ray beam 10 cm ventral to the rostral third of the facial crest.
8. Collimate around the area of interest.
9. Exposure guide: 77 kVp, 20 mAs.

Open-mouth Right 10° dorsal-left ventral oblique (R10D-LVO) and Left 10° dorsal-right ventral oblique (L10D-RVO) (Fig. 14.31)

1. Keep the mouth open with a gag that leaves the cheek teeth free.
2. Place the plate on the affected side in a vertical position and orientated to the area of interest.

   – R10D-LVO: outlines the left-sided mandibular cheek teeth erupted crown.
   – L10D-RVO: outlines the right-sided mandibular cheek teeth erupted crown.

3. Indicate right/left (plate's side) with a marker.
4. Position the X-ray machine on the contralateral side of the head.
5. Focus–film distance: 100 cm.
6. Angle the X-ray beam, so that the X-ray beam hits the dorsal plane (hard palate) at a 10-degree downward angle.
7. Centre the X-ray beam at the level of the rostral third of the facial crest.
8. Collimate around the area of interest.
9. Exposure guide: 77 kVp, 20 mAs.

A

R15V-LDO
Dorsal

Right
Lateral ⤒ 15°

Left
Lateral

Ventral

B

R10D-LVO
Dorsal

Right
Lateral

Left
Lateral

⤒ 10°

Ventral

C

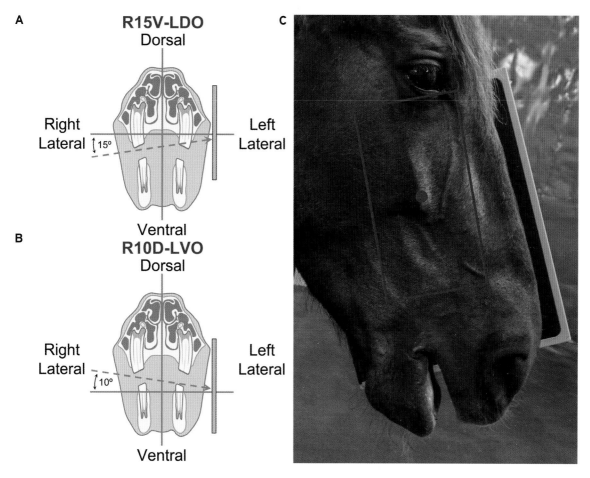

Figure 14.31 Diagram (A and B) and positioning (C) to obtain both open-mouth R15V-LDO (A) and R10D-LVO (B) views of the head for the left-sided maxillary and mandibular cheek teeth erupted crown, respectively.

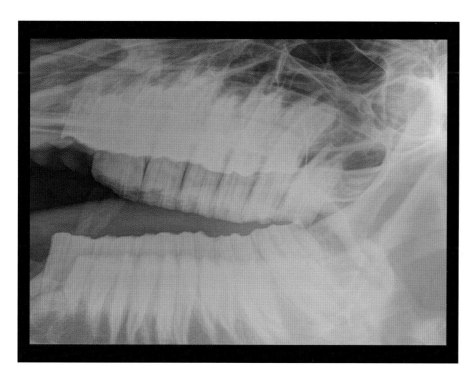

Figure 14.32
Open-mouth R15V-LDO projection of the head that outlines the left-sided maxillary cheek teeth erupted crown.

Rostro 35° latero 50° ventral-caudodorsal oblique (R35L50V-CdDO) (Figs 14.33–14.36)

1. Position the head horizontal to the ground with the help of a head stand. Avoid any tilting or rotation of the head.
2. Place the plate in horizontal position facing downwards dorsal to the head, above the poll region.
3. Indicate right/left with a marker.
4. Position the X-ray machine below and to the side of the area to be examined, at a 35-degree angle from the sagittal plane of the head.
5. Focus–film distance: 100 cm.
6. Angle the X-ray beam, so that the X-ray beam hits the dorsal plane (hard palate) at a 50-degree upward angle.
7. Centre the X-ray beam at the level of the temporomandibular joint.
8. Collimate around the area of interest.
9. Exposure guide: 75 kVp, 30 mAs.

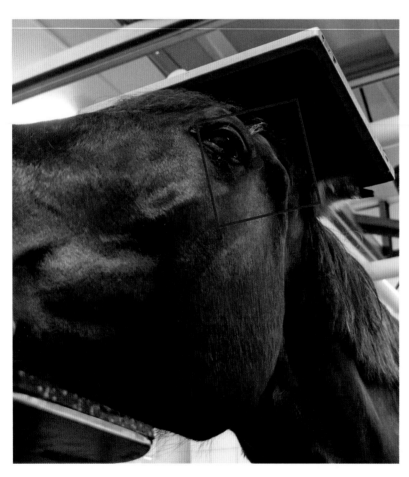

Figure 14.33 Positioning to obtain an R35L50V-CdDO view of the temporomandibular joint.

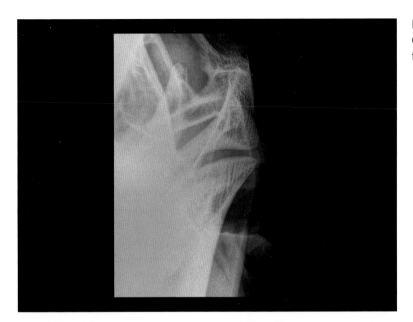

Figure 14.34 R35L50V-CdDO projection of the temporomandibular joint.

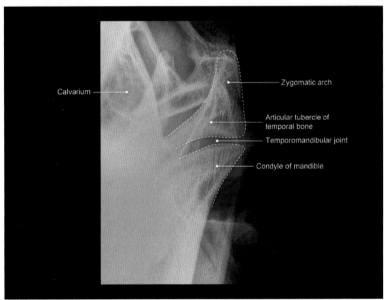

Calvarium

Zygomatic arch

Articular tubercle of temporal bone

Temporomandibular joint

Condyle of mandible

Figure 14.35 Radiographic anatomy of the R35L50V-CdDO projection of the temporomandibular joint.

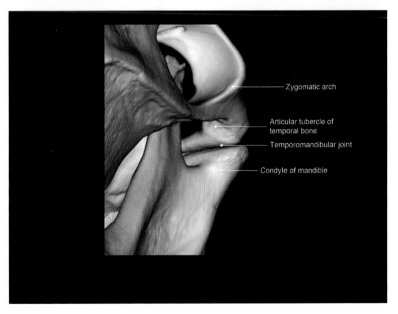

Zygomatic arch

Articular tubercle of temporal bone

Temporomandibular joint

Condyle of mandible

Figure 14.36 3D representation of the R35L50V-CdDO projection of the temporomandibular joint.

CHAPTER 15

Cervical spine

Indications

Radiography of the cervical spine is becoming more and more common and is useful in the diagnosis of horses with:

- Ataxia and abnormal gait
- Neck pain and stiffness
- Cervical trauma
- Abnormal head or neck carriage
- Forelimb lameness unable to localize by diagnostic analgesia
- Scintigraphic or ultrasonographic findings suggestive of cervical disease
- Non-specific signs of neck problems including: poor performance and equitation problems
- As part of a pre-purchase examination.

Equipment

For a complete study of the cervical spine, the following equipment is required:

- Portable X-ray machine is sufficient for the cranial and mid neck; more caudal projections require a high-output generator
- Large plates (35 × 43 cm)
- Parallel grid, depending on the system used
- Rope/webbing headcollar to avoid metal artefacts in the cranial neck region
- Blinkers
- Head stand
- Mounted plate holder (ceiling- or wall-mounted)
- Radiation safety equipment: lead gowns and thyroid protectors.

Preparation

Sedation of the patient is advised. The use of blinkers is helpful in some cases.

Radiographic protocol

A standard radiographic examination of the cervical spine of an adult horse is composed of four overlapping laterolateral (LL) views.
Additional projections:

- Ventrodorsal (VD) of the cranial neck
- Right ventral-left dorsal oblique (RV-LDO) and left ventral-right dorsal oblique (LV-RDO).

Laterolateral (LL) (Figs 15.1–15.13)

1. Stand the horse square with all limbs equally weight-bearing and extend the neck slightly with the help of a head stand. Avoid any tilting or rotation of the head and neck. When obtaining radiographs of the cranial neck and occiput it may be useful to use a rope/webbing headcollar and to pull the ears forward by attaching tape. Elevating the head and neck may facilitate imaging the caudal portion of the neck.

2. Place the plate on one side of the neck in a vertical position in landscape orientation.

3. Indicate right/left (plate's side) with a marker.

4. Position the X-ray machine on the other side of the neck.

5. Focus–film distance: 100 cm. If a grid is used, adjust the focus–film distance to the distance specified for the grid.

6. Use a horizontal X-ray beam, perpendicular to the long axis of the neck and the plate.

7. Centre the X-ray beam dorsal to the jugular groove; the level depends on the area of interest:

   – Cranial neck: wings of the atlas
   – Mid neck: C3
   – Caudal neck: C5
   – Cervicothoracic junction: C7.

8. It is helpful to palpate the neck and use tape to mark position of the plate/centring. Beware that some tape is radiodense though and shows up on the radiograph!

9. Align the field of view with the long axis of the cervical spine and collimate around the area of interest.

10. Exposure guide:

    – Cranial neck: 70 kVp, 20 mAs
    – Mid neck: 80 kVp, 30 mAs
    – Caudal neck: 85 kVp, 40 mAs
    – Cervicothoracic junction: 95 kVp, 60 mAs.

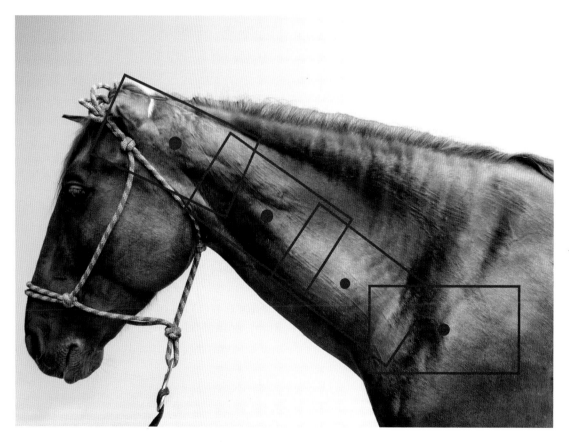

Figure 15.1 Positioning to obtain LL views of the cervical spine.

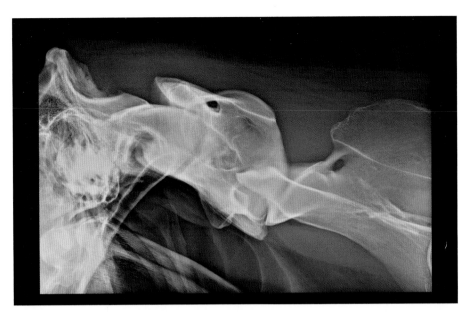

Figure 15.2
LL projection of the cranial portion of the cervical spine.

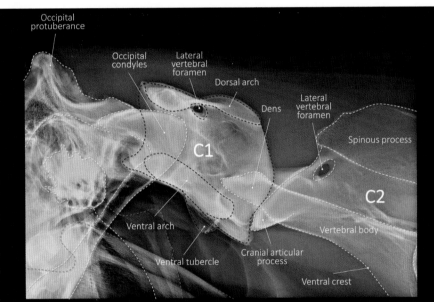

Figure 15.3
Radiographic anatomy of the LL projection of the cranial portion of the cervical spine.

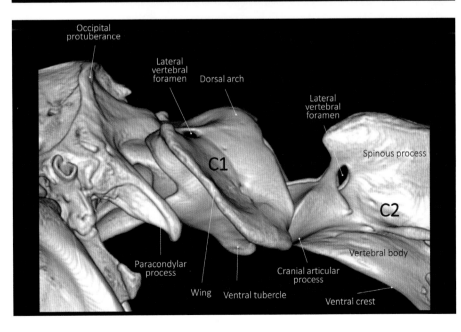

Figure 15.4
3D representation of the LL projection of the cranial portion of the cervical spine.

Figure 15.5
LL projection of the mid portion of the cervical spine.

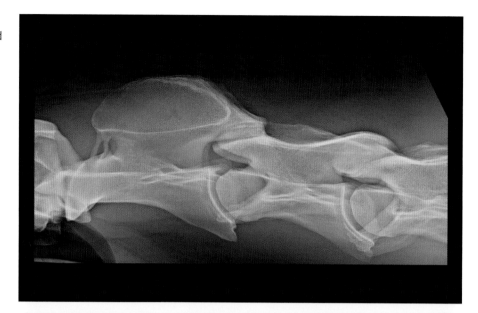

Figure 15.6
Radiographic anatomy of the LL projection of the mid portion of the cervical spine.

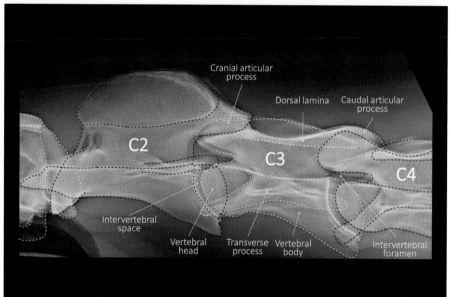

Figure 15.7
3D representation of the LL projection of the mid portion of the cervical spine.

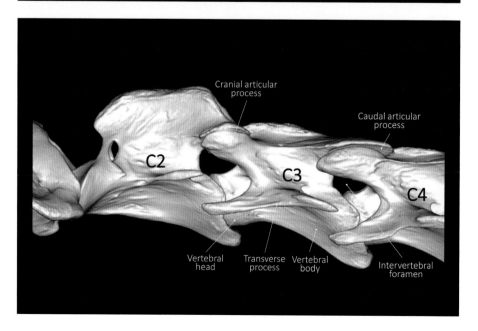

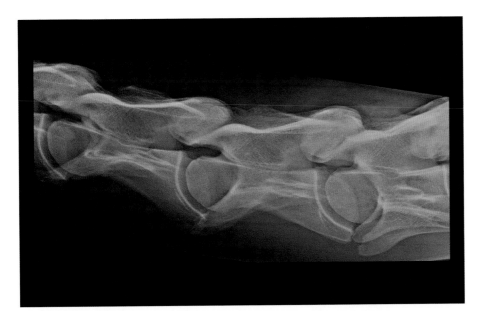

Figure 15.8
LL projection of the caudal portion of the cervical spine.

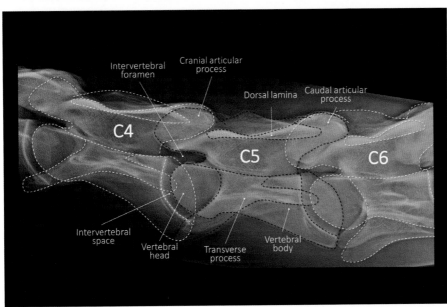

Figure 15.9
Radiographic anatomy of the LL projection of the caudal portion of the cervical spine.

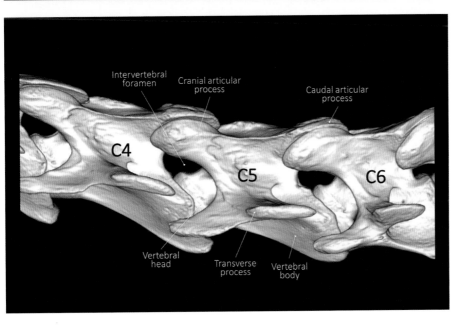

Figure 15.10
3D representation of the LL projection of the caudal portion of the cervical spine.

Figure 15.11
LL projection of
the cervicothoracic
junction.

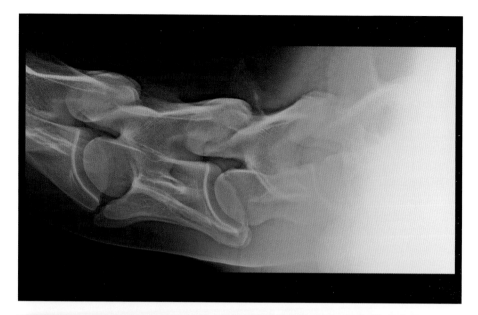

Figure 15.12
Radiographic anatomy
of the LL projection
of the cervicothoracic
junction.

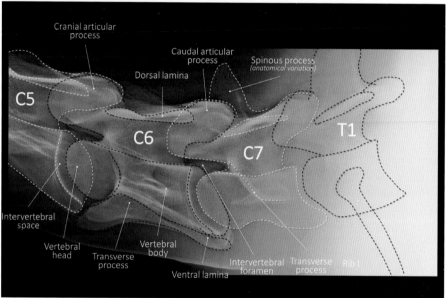

Figure 15.13
3D representation of
the LL projection of
the cervicothoracic
junction.

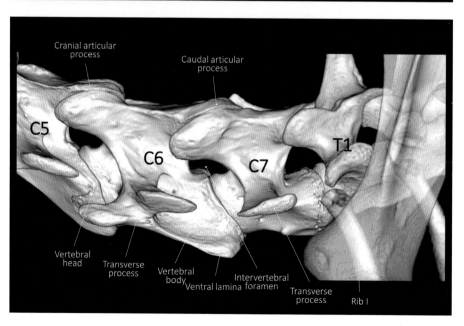

Ventrodorsal (VD) of the cranial neck (Figs 15.14–15.16)

1. Extend the head and neck by positioning the head horizontal to the ground with the help of a head stand. Avoid any tilting or rotation of the head and neck.
2. Place the plate horizontally facing downward on the dorsal side of the cranial aspect of the neck.
3. Indicate right/left with a marker.
4. Position the X-ray machine ventral to the cranial aspect of the neck.
5. Focus–film distance: 100 cm. If a grid is used, adjust the focus–film distance to the distance specified for the grid.
6. Orientate the X-ray beam obliquely upwards, perpendicular to the plate.
7. Centre the X-ray beam in the midline of the cranial neck, at the level of the wings of the atlas.
8. Collimate around the area of interest.
9. Exposure guide: 90 kVp, 55 mAs.

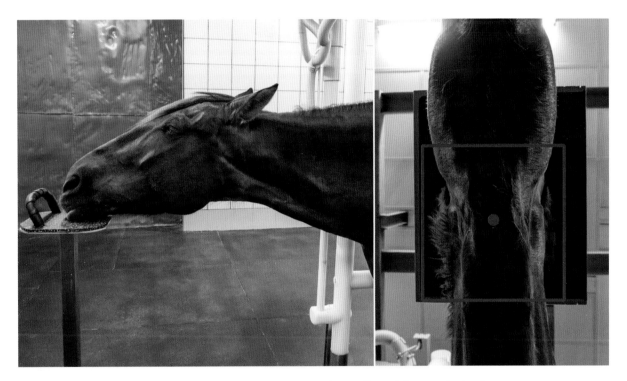

Figure 15.14 Positioning to obtain a VD view of the cranial portion of the cervical spine.

Figure 15.15
VD projection of the cranial portion of the cervical spine.

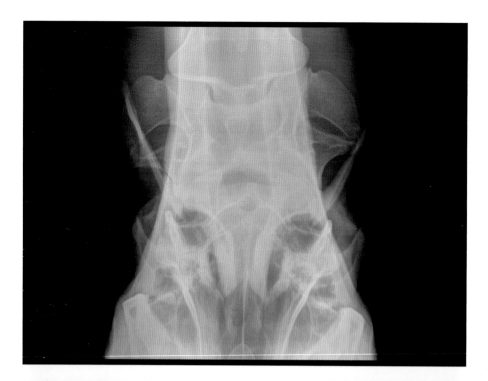

Figure 15.16
Radiographic anatomy of the VD projection of the cranial portion of the cervical spine.

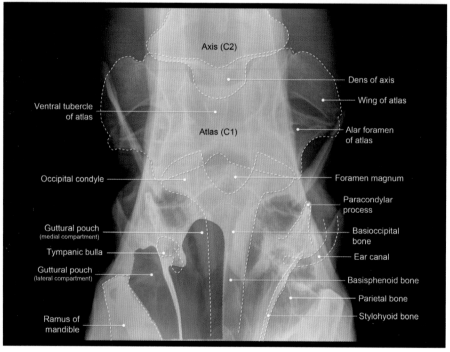

Right ventral-left dorsal oblique (RV-LDO) and left ventral-right dorsal oblique (LV-RDO) for articular process ('facet') joints (Figs 15.17–15.26)

1. Stand the horse square with all limbs equally weight-bearing and extend the neck slightly with the help of a head stand. Avoid any tilting or rotation of the head and neck.
2. Place the plate on the dorsolateral side of the neck in landscape orientation, perpendicular to the X-ray beam. Beware that this may be higher than you think!
3. Indicate right/left (plate's side) with a marker.
4. Position the X-ray machine on the ventro-lateral aspect of the contralateral side of the neck.

   - RV-LDO: outlines the right-sided articular processes in an 'end-on' view and the left-sided articular process joints' articular spaces.
   - LV-RDO: outlines the left-sided articular processes in an 'end-on' view and the right-sided articular process joints' articular spaces.

   Note: this is the opposite way in the back due to the different orientation of the articular process joints.

5. Focus–film distance: 100 cm. If a grid is used, adjust the focus–film distance to the distance specified for the grid.
6. Angle the X-ray beam upwards 45–55 degrees from the horizontal, perpendicular to the long axis of the neck. The articular process joints change their angulation from cranial to caudal requiring a shallower angle cranially and a steeper angle caudally.
7. Centre the X-ray beam at the jugular groove. The level depends on the area of interest:

   - Cranial neck: C1–C2
   - Mid neck: C3–C4
   - Caudal neck: C5–C6.

   It is helpful to palpate the neck and use tape to mark position of the plate/centring. Beware that some tape is radiodense though and shows up on the radiograph!

8. Align the field of view with the long axis of the cervical spine and collimate around the area of interest.
9. Exposure guide:

   - Cranial neck: 70 kVp, 20 mAs
   - Mid neck: 80 kVp, 30 mAs
   - Caudal neck: 85 kVp, 55 mAs.

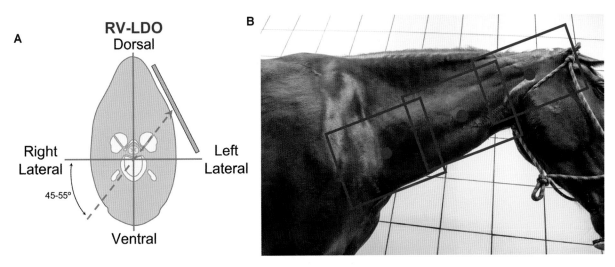

Figure 15.17 Diagram (A) and positioning (B) to obtain an RV-LDO view of the cervical spine that outlines the right-sided articular processes in an 'end-on' view and the left-sided articular process joints' articular spaces.

Figure 15.18 RV-LDO projection of the cranial portion of the cervical spine, outlines the right-sided articular processes in an 'end-on' view and the left-sided articular process joints' articular spaces.

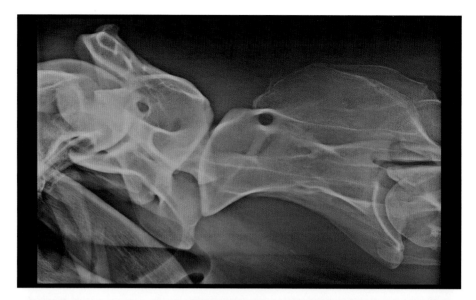

Figure 15.19 Radiographic anatomy of the RV-LDO projection of the cranial portion of the cervical spine, outlines the right-sided articular processes in an 'end-on' view and the left-sided articular process joints' articular spaces.

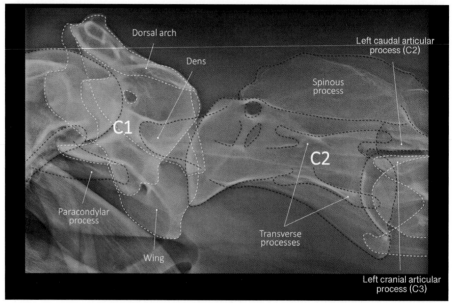

Figure 15.20 3D representation of the RV-LDO projection of the cranial portion of the cervical spine, outlines the right-sided articular processes in an 'end-on' view and the left-sided articular process joints' articular spaces.

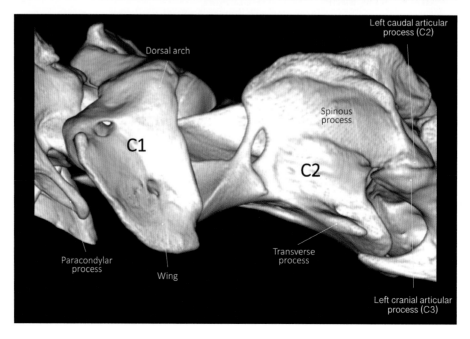

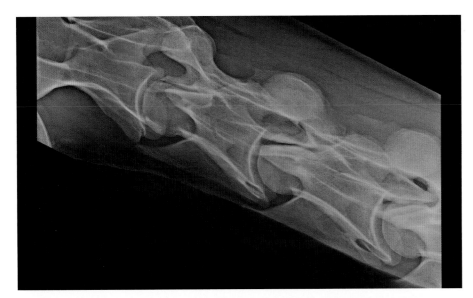

Figure 15.21 RV-LDO projection of the mid portion of the cervical spine, outlines the right-sided articular processes in an 'end-on' view and the left-sided articular process joints' articular spaces.

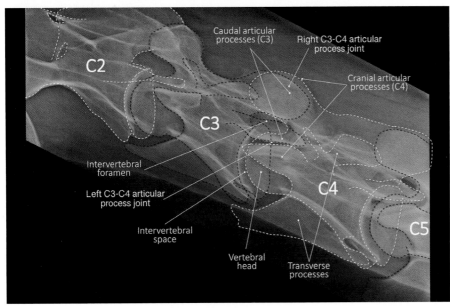

Figure 15.22 Radiographic anatomy of the RV-LDO projection of the mid portion of the cervical spine, outlines the right-sided articular processes in an 'end-on' view and the left-sided articular process joints' articular spaces.

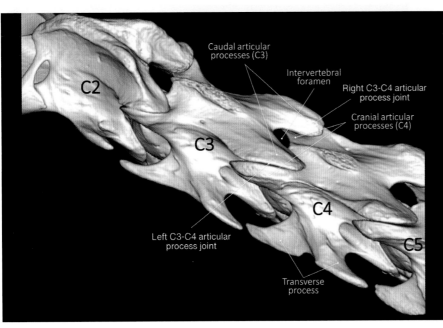

Figure 15.23 3D representation of the RV-LDO projection of the mid portion of the cervical spine, outlines the right-sided articular processes in an 'end-on' view and the left-sided articular process joints' articular spaces.

Figure 15.24 RV-LDO projection of the caudal portion of the cervical spine, outlines the right-sided articular processes in an 'end-on' view and the left-sided articular process joints' articular spaces.

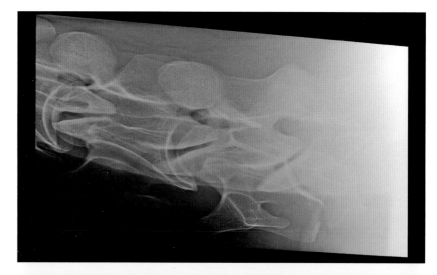

Figure 15.25 Radiographic anatomy of the RV-LDO projection of the caudal portion of the cervical spine, outlines the right-sided articular processes in an 'end-on' view and the left-sided articular process joints' articular spaces.

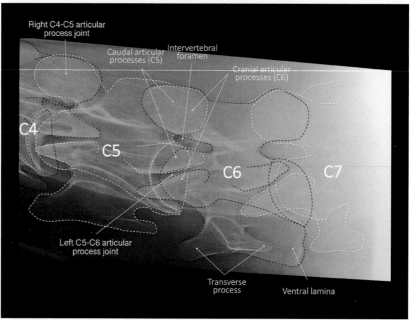

Figure 15.26 3D representation of the RV-LDO projection of the caudal portion of the cervical spine, outlines the right-sided articular processes in an 'end-on' view and the left-sided articular process joints' articular spaces.

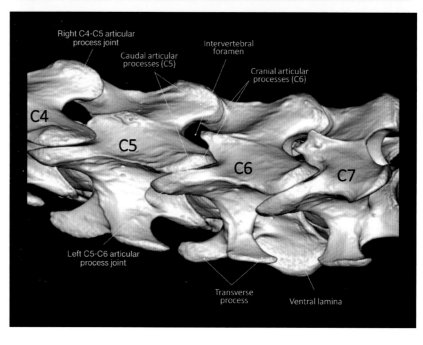

CHAPTER 16

Back

Indications

Radiography of the thoracolumbar spine is nowadays a common diagnostic procedure, especially in performance horses. Quality radiographs of this region are useful in the diagnosis of horses with:

- Back pain and stiffness
- Thoracolumbar trauma
- Ataxia and abnormal gait
- Positive response to regional analgesia
- Hind limb lameness that cannot be localized to other anatomical regions by diagnostic analgesia
- Scintigraphic findings suggestive of thoracolumbar disease
- Non-specific clinical signs including poor performance and equitation problems
- As part of a pre-purchase examination.

Equipment

For a complete study of the thoracolumbar spine the following equipment is required:

- Portable X-ray machine is sufficient for thoracic spinous processes. High-output generator may be necessary for vertebral bodies, articular process joints and lumbar spine

- Large plates (35 × 43 cm)
- Parallel grid, depending on system used
- Aluminium wedge or silicon wedge to level out discrepancy in radiodensities caused by the different thickness of the spine
- Sheet of lead
- Blinkers
- Head stand
- Mounted plate holder (ceiling- or wall-mounted)
- Radiation safety equipment: lead gowns and thyroid protectors.

Preparation

Sedation of the patient is advised. The use of blinkers may be helpful. Divide the back according to the size of the plate so each view overlaps slightly. This is achieved by placing radiopaque markers along the thoracolumbar spine, which will also enable the identification of specific vertebrae on the radiographs. Beware that markers (especially if they are very radiodense or big) may affect the processing of the image and cause artefacts. In standard adult horses, four markers are usually enough when using large plates (Fig. 16.1):

- First marker: withers (T6)
- Second marker: mid thoracic spine (T11–T12)

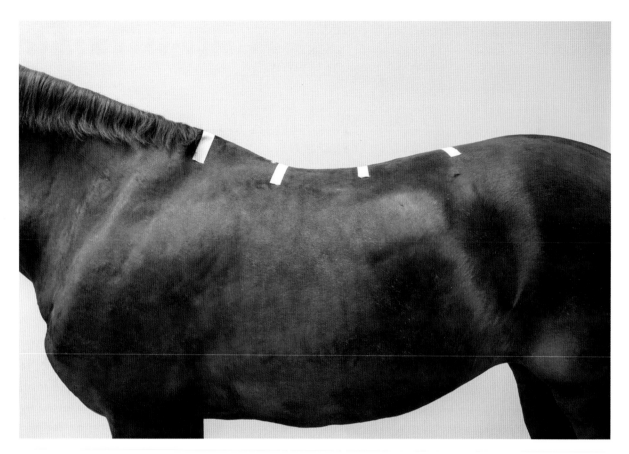

Figure 16.1 Positioning of the markers along the thoracolumbar spine.

• Third marker: thoracolumbar junction (T18–L1)
• Fourth marker: mid lumbar spine (L3).

Marker placement is helped by either palpating cranially from the lumbosacral junction which can be felt as a dip or from the last (18th) rib.

Radiographic protocol
A standard radiographic examination of the thoracolumbar spine of an adult horse comprises a series of several overlapping laterolateral (LL) views for the spinous processes and a separate series for the vertebral bodies.

Additional oblique projections are acquired to separate the left and right articular process ('facet') joints:

• Right 20° ventral-left dorsal oblique (R20V-LDO) and Left 20° ventral-right dorsal oblique (L20V-RDO).

Laterolateral (LL) of the spinous processes (Figs 16.2–16.21)

1. Stand the horse square with all limbs equally weight-bearing with the neck in neutral position and the head resting on a head stand. Avoid any rotation or tilting of the trunk. Standardization of the neck position is advisable since neck position affects the width of the interspinous spaces, one of the parameters evaluated for 'kissing spines'.

2. An aluminium wedge can be placed on the plate's side of the trunk to compensate for the different thickness of overlying soft tissues. Alternatively, a silicon wedge can be used that is placed in front of the X-ray machine to achieve the same effect. These are used in human shoulder radiography and can usually be purchased through a human hospital supplier.

3. Place the plate on one side of the trunk in a vertical position in landscape orientation.

4. Indicate right/left (plate's side) with a marker.

5. Position the X-ray machine on the other side of the body.

6. Focus–film distance: 120 cm. If a grid is used, adjust the focus–film distance to the distance specified for the grid.

7. Use a horizontal X-ray beam, perpendicular to the long axis of the thoracolumbar spine.

8. Centre the X-ray beam approximately 10 cm ventral to the dorsal outline of the back using these markers as a reference:

   – Cranial thoracic spinous processes: first marker (Fig. 16.2)
   – Mid thoracic spinous processes: between first and second marker (Fig. 16.3)
   – Caudal thoracic spinous processes: between second and third marker (Fig. 16.4)
   – Cranial lumbar spinous processes: between third and fourth marker (Fig. 16.5)
   – Caudal lumbar spinous processes: fourth marker (Fig. 16.6).

9. Align the field of view with the long axis of the thoracolumbar spine and collimate around the area of interest.

10. Exposure guide:

    – Cranial thoracic spine: 80 kVp, 30 mAs
    – Mid thoracic spine: 65 kVp, 20 mAs
    – Caudal thoracic spine: 85 kVp, 35 mAs
    – Lumbar spine: 90 kVp, 40 mAs.

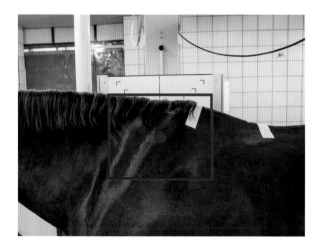

Figure 16.2 Positioning to obtain a LL view of the cranial thoracic spinous processes.

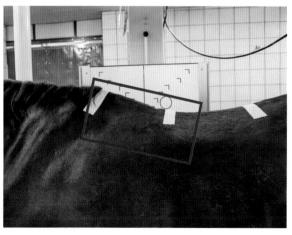

Figure 16.3 Positioning to obtain a LL view of the mid thoracic spinous processes.

Figure 16.4 Positioning to obtain a LL view of the caudal thoracic spinous processes.

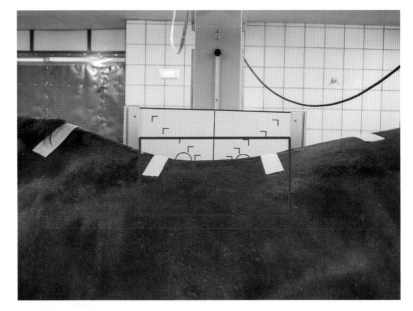

Figure 16.5 Positioning to obtain a LL view of the cranial lumbar spinous processes.

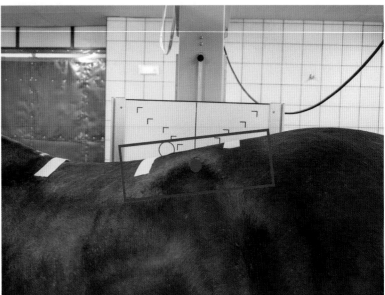

Figure 16.6 Positioning to obtain a LL view of the caudal lumbar spinous processes.

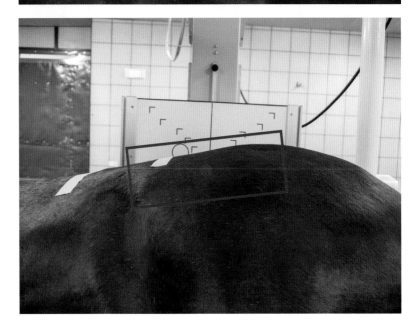

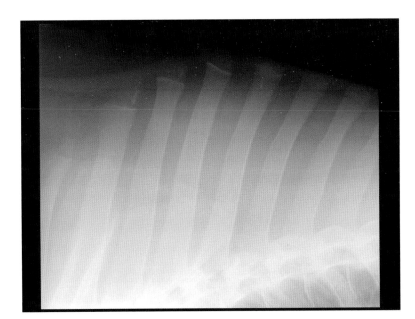

Figure 16.7 LL projection of the cranial thoracic spinous processes.

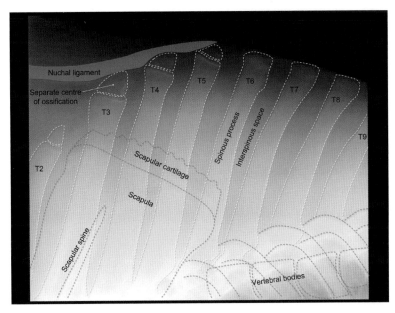

Figure 16.8 Radiographic anatomy of the LL projection of the cranial thoracic spinous processes.

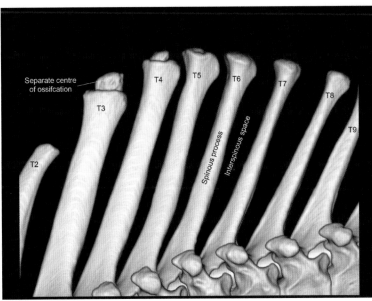

Figure 16.9 3D representation of the LL projection of the cranial thoracic spinous processes.

Figure 16.10 LL projection of the mid thoracic spinous processes.

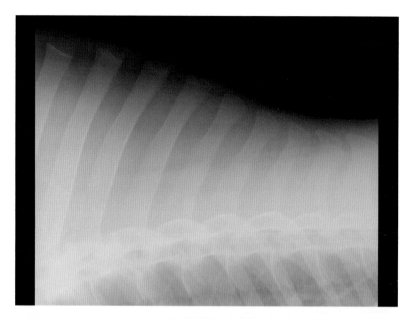

Figure 16.11 Radiographic anatomy of the LL projection of the mid thoracic spinous processes.

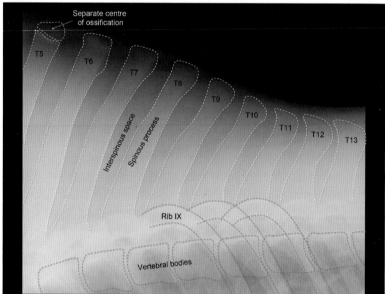

Figure 16.12 3D representation of the LL projection of the mid thoracic spinous processes.

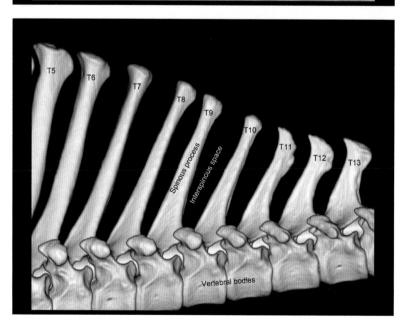

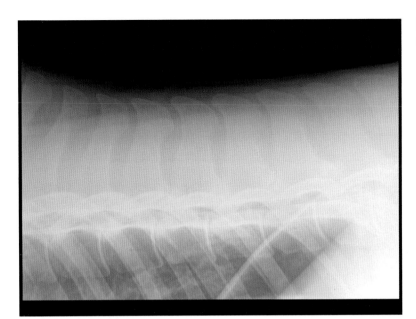

Figure 16.13 LL projection of the caudal thoracic spinous processes.

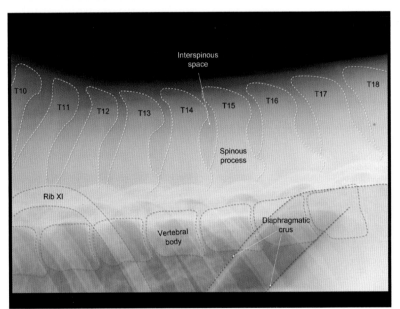

Figure 16.14 Radiographic anatomy of the LL projection of the caudal thoracic spinous processes.

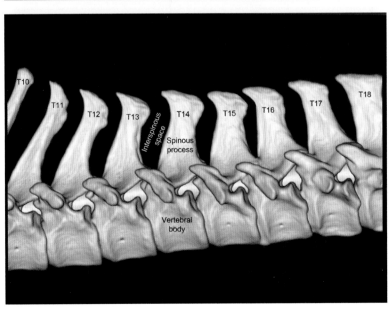

Figure 16.15 3D representation of the LL projection of the caudal thoracic spinous processes.

Figure 16.16 LL projection of the cranial lumbar spinous processes.

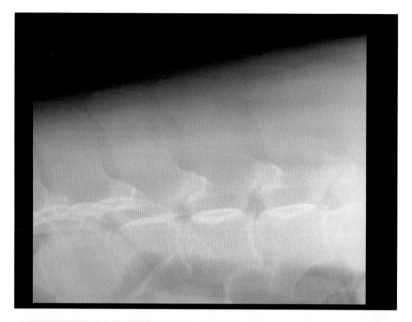

Figure 16.17 Radiographic anatomy of the LL projection of the cranial lumbar spinous processes.

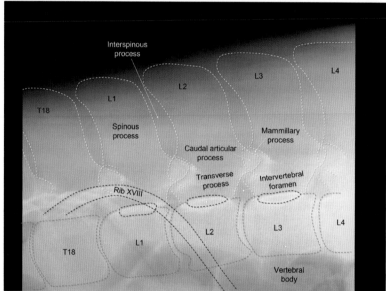

Figure 16.18 3D representation of the LL projection of the cranial lumbar spinous processes.

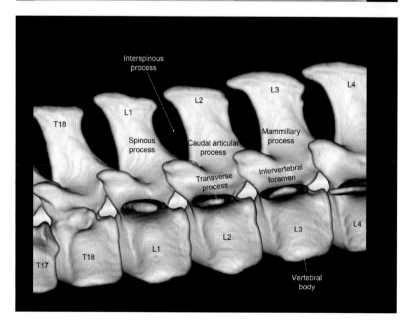

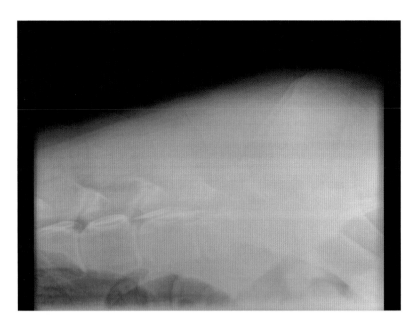

Figure 16.19 LL projection of the caudal lumbar spinous processes.

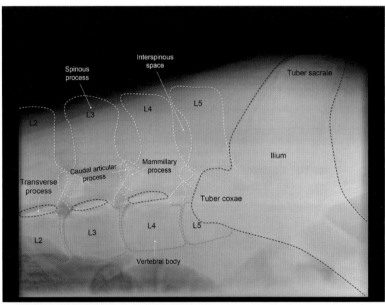

Figure 16.20 Radiographic anatomy of the LL projection of the caudal lumbar spinous processes.

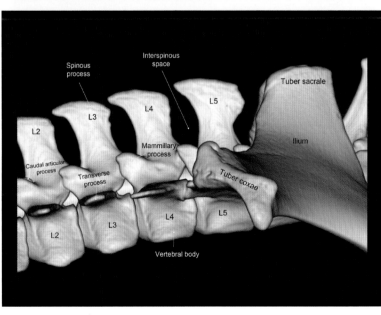

Figure 16.21 3D representation of the LL projection of the caudal lumbar spinous processes.

Laterolateral (LL) of the vertebral bodies (Figs 16.22–16.37)

1. Stand the horse square with all limbs equally weight-bearing with the neck in neutral position and the head resting on a head stand. Avoid any rotation or tilting of the trunk. When radiographing the lumbar vertebral bodies, a sheet of lead can be placed onto the skin surface of the lumbar region in order to reduce the scatter.
2. Place the plate on one side of the trunk in a vertical position in landscape orientation.
3. Indicate right/left (plate's side) with a marker.
4. Position the X-ray machine on the other side of the body.
5. Focus–film distance: 120 cm. If a grid is used, adjust the focus–film distance to the distance specified for the grid.
6. Use a horizontal X-ray beam, perpendicular to the long axis of the thoracolumbar spine.

7. Centre the X-ray beam approximately 15–20 cm ventral to the dorsal outline of the back using these markers as a reference:

   – Cranial thoracic vertebral bodies: first marker (Fig. 16.22).
   – Mid thoracic vertebral bodies: between first and second marker (Fig. 16.23).
   – Caudal thoracic vertebral bodies: between second and third marker (Fig. 16.24).
   – Lumbar vertebral bodies: between third and fourth marker (Fig. 16.25).

8. Align the field of view with the long axis of the thoracolumbar spine and collimate around the area of interest.
9. Exposure guide:

   – Thoracic spine: 100 kVp, 50 mAs
   – Lumbar spine: 120 kVp, 100 mAs.

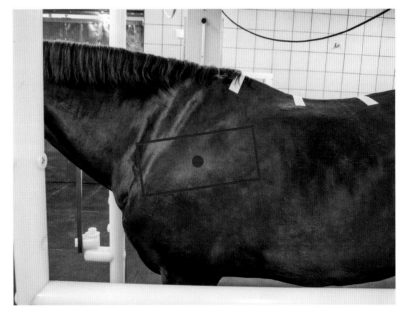

Figure 16.22 Positioning to obtain a LL view of the cranial thoracic vertebral bodies.

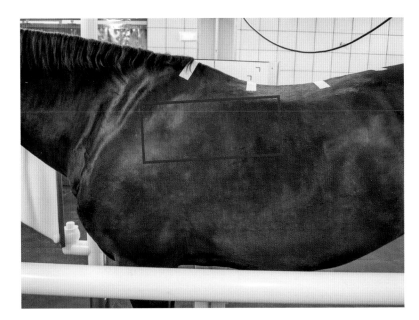

Figure 16.23 Positioning to obtain a LL view of the mid thoracic vertebral bodies.

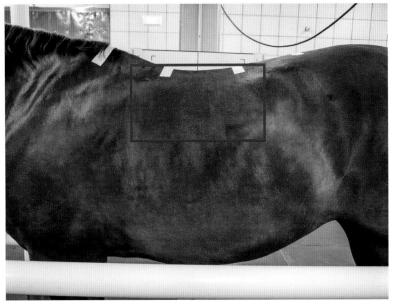

Figure 16.24 Positioning to obtain a LL view of the caudal thoracic vertebral bodies.

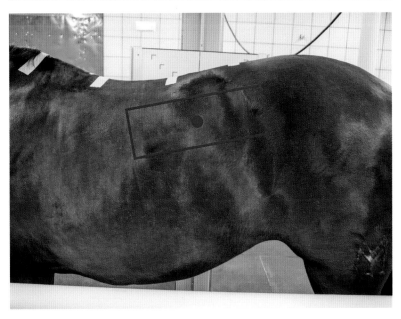

Figure 16.25 Positioning to obtain a LL view of the lumbar vertebral bodies.

Figure 16.26 LL projection of the cranial thoracic vertebral bodies.

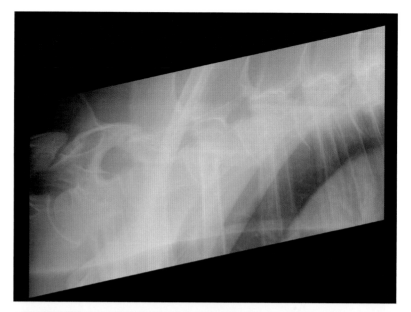

Figure 16.27 Radiographic anatomy of the LL projection of the cranial thoracic vertebral bodies.

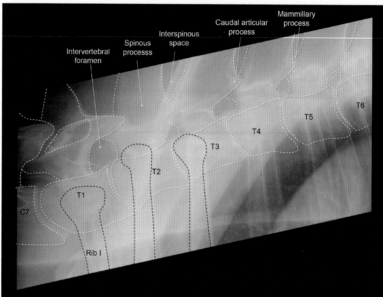

Figure 16.28 3D representation of the LL projection of the cranial thoracic vertebral bodies.

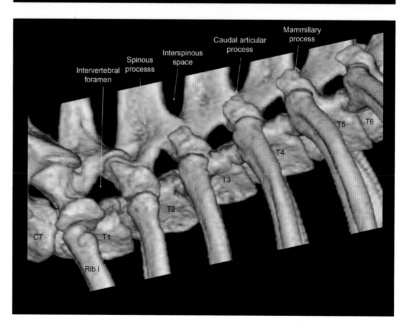

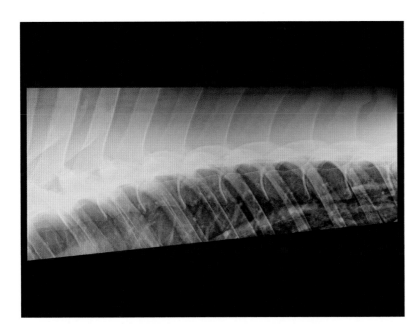

Figure 16.29 LL projection of the mid thoracic vertebral bodies.

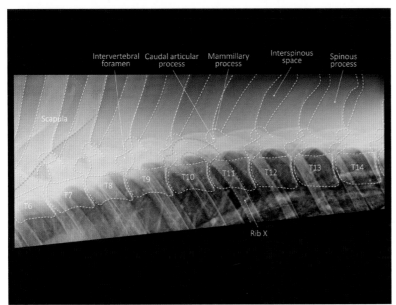

Figure 16.30 Radiographic anatomy of the LL projection of the mid thoracic vertebral bodies.

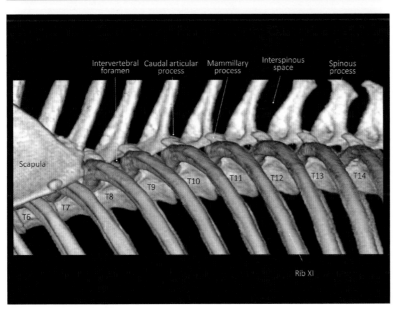

Figure 16.31 3D representation of the LL projection of the mid thoracic vertebral bodies.

Figure 16.32 LL projection of the caudal thoracic vertebral bodies.

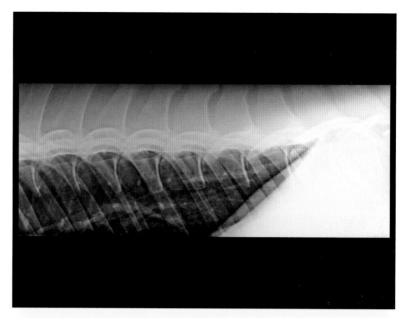

Figure 16.33 Radiographic anatomy of the LL projection of the caudal thoracic vertebral bodies.

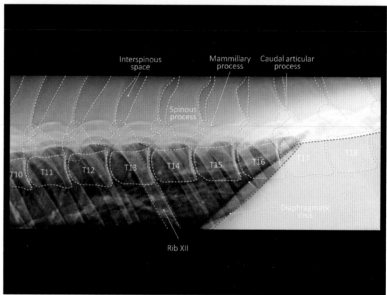

Figure 16.34 3D representation of the LL projection of the caudal thoracic vertebral bodies.

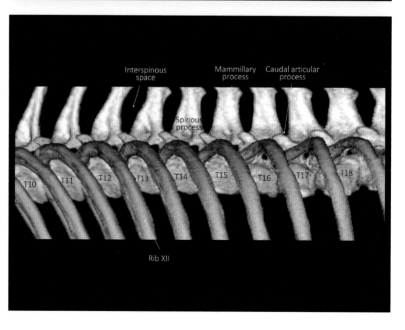

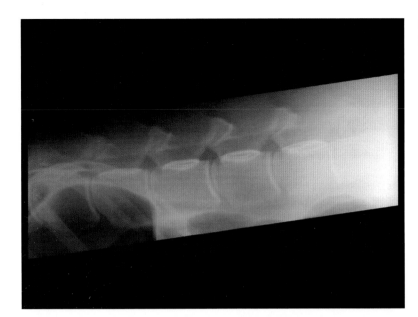

Figure 16.35 LL projection of the lumbar vertebral bodies.

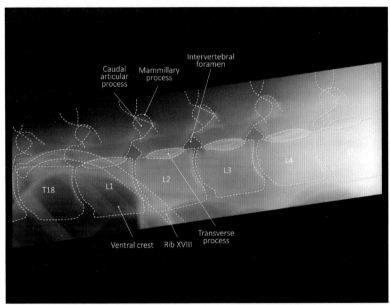

Figure 16.36 Radiographic anatomy of the LL projection of the lumbar vertebral bodies.

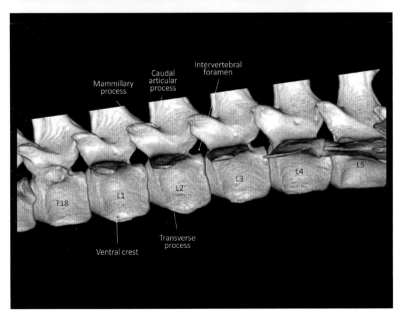

Figure 16.37 3D representation of the LL projection of the lumbar vertebral bodies.

Right 20° ventral-left dorsal oblique (R20V-LDO) and left 20° ventral-right dorsal oblique (L20V-RDO)
(Figs 16.38-16.41)

1. Stand the horse square with all limbs equally weight-bearing with the neck in neutral position and the head resting on a head stand. Avoid any rotation or tilting of the trunk.
2. Place the plate on the dorsolateral side of the trunk in landscape orientation on the contralateral side of the joint of interest.
3. Indicate right/left (plate's side) with a marker.
4. Position the X-ray machine on the ventrolateral aspect of the trunk on the side of the joint of interest. Usually one would acquire radiographs from both sides.

   - R20V-LDO: outlines the right-sided articular process joints.
   - L20V-RDO: outlines the left-sided articular process joints.

Note: this is the opposite way in the neck due to the different orientation of the articular process joints.

5. Focus–film distance: 120 cm. If a grid is used, adjust the focus–film distance to the distance specified for the grid.
6. Angle the X-ray beam 20 degrees upwards from the horizontal, perpendicular to the long axis of the thoracolumbar spine.
7. Centre the X-ray beam approximately 20–25 cm ventral to the dorsal outline of the back using these markers as a reference:

   - Mid thoracic articular process joints: between first and second marker
   - Caudal thoracic articular process joints: between second and third marker.

8. Align the field of view with the long axis of the thoracolumbar spine and collimate around the area of interest.
9. Exposure guide: 100 kVp, 40 mAs.

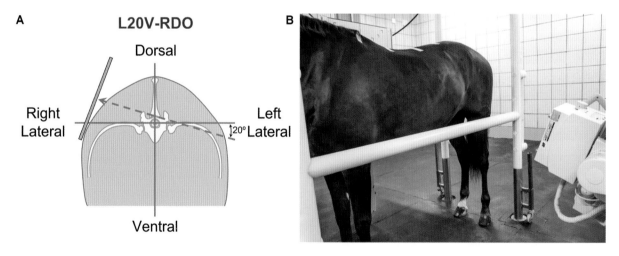

Figure 16.38 Diagram (A) and positioning (B) to obtain an L20V-RDO view of the caudal thoracic spine that outlines the left-sided articular process joints.

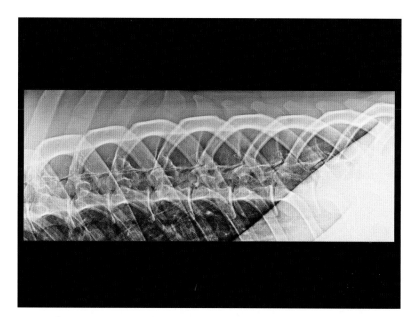

Figure 16.39 L2OV-RDO projection of the caudal thoracic spine outlines the left-sided articular process joints.

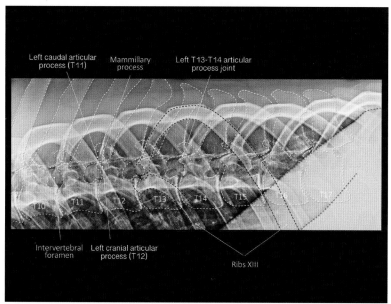

Figure 16.40 Radiographic anatomy of the L2OV-RDO projection of the caudal thoracic spine outlines the left-sided articular process joints.

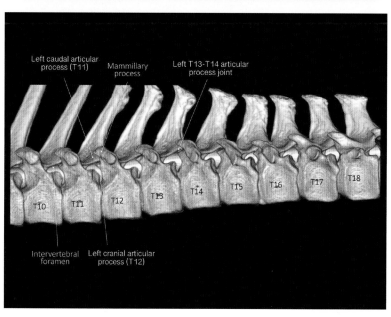

Figure 16.41 3D representation of the L2OV-RDO projection of the caudal thoracic spine outlines the left-sided articular process joints.

CHAPTER 17

Thorax

Indications

Radiography of the thorax in a full-sized, adult horse requires high exposures and is usually reserved to referral centres. Main indications for obtaining thoracic radiographs are:

- Clinical signs of lower respiratory or cardiac disease: cough, bilateral nasal discharge, tachypnoea and dyspnoea
- Abnormal lung sounds
- Exercise intolerance
- Fever of unknown origin
- Further evaluation of abnormal ultrasonographic findings.

Equipment

For a complete study of the thorax the following equipment is required:

- High-output X-ray generator
- Large plates (35 × 43 cm)
- Parallel grid depending on the system
- Blinkers may be helpful
- Mounted plate holder (ceiling- or wall-mounted)
- Radiation safety equipment: lead gowns, lead gloves and thyroid protectors.

Preparation

Sedation of the patient is advised. The use of blinkers is also helpful.

Divide the thorax according to the size of the plates so each view overlaps slightly. In the standard adult horse, the thorax is divided into four quadrants by delineating two perpendicular lines, a vertical one extending caudodorsally from the olecranon and a horizontal one extending caudally from the shoulder (Fig. 17.1):

- Craniodorsal
- Cranioventral
- Caudodorsal
- Caudoventral.

Note: in some horses, it may be helpful to use auscultation or percussion to delineate the lung field!

Radiographic protocol

A standard radiographic examination of the thorax of an adult horse is composed of four overlapping laterolateral (LL) views. In ponies and small horses one or two views may be sufficient to cover the whole lung field. The radiographs should be obtained in full inspiration. Foals can be radiographed either in lateral recumbency or standing.

Additional projections that can be obtained in foals:

- Ventrodorsal (VD).

Laterolateral (LL) standing in adult horses (Figs 17.1–17.9)

1. Stand the horse square with all limbs equally weight-bearing. Avoid any rotation or tilting of the body.
2. Place the plate on one side of the thorax in a vertical position in landscape orientation, except for the cranioventral projection, where the plate is usually placed in portrait orientation.
3. Indicate right/left (plate's side) with a marker.
4. Position the X-ray machine on the other side of the body.
5. Focus–film distance: 120 cm. If a grid is used, adjust the focus–film distance to the distance specified for the grid.
6. Use a horizontal X-ray beam, perpendicular to the long axis of the trunk.
7. X-ray centring depends on the quadrant (Fig. 17.1):

   – Craniodorsal: in the dorsal third of a line between the most caudal aspect of the scapula and the olecranon or in the dorsal third of the 4th intercostal space
   – Cranioventral: 10 cm caudal to the shoulder joint or in the middle third of the 2nd–3rd intercostal spaces
   – Caudodorsal: in the dorsal third of the 11th intercostal space
   – Caudoventral: in the middle third of the 6th–7th intercostal spaces.

8. Collimate to the edge of the plate.
9. Exposure guide:

   – Craniodorsal and caudoventral: 80 kVp, 30 mAs
   – Cranioventral: 110 kVp, 50 mAs
   – Caudoventral: 90 kVp, 40 mAs.

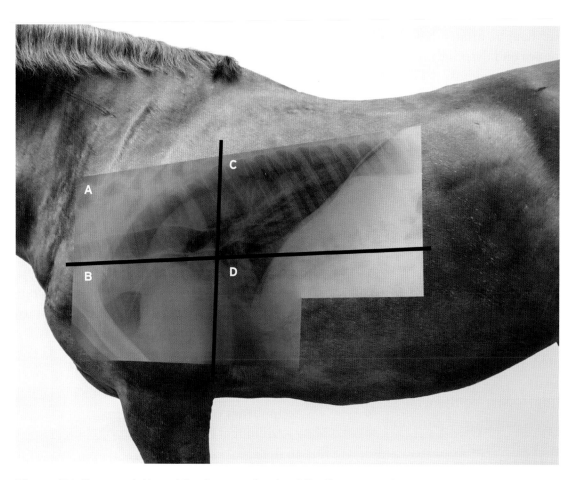

Figure 17.1 Representation of the four quadrants of the thorax: craniodorsal (A), cranioventral (B), caudodorsal (C) and caudoventral (D).

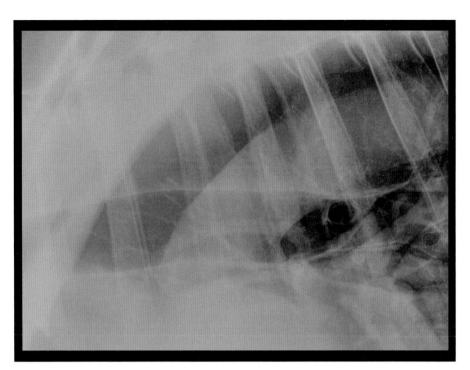

Figure 17.2
LL projection of the craniodorsal quadrant of the thorax.

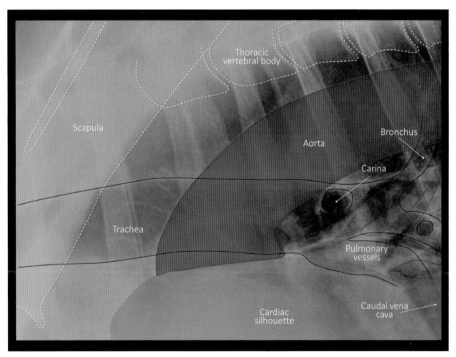

Figure 17.3
Radiographic anatomy of the LL projection of the craniodorsal quadrant of the thorax.

Figure 17.4
LL projection of the
cranioventral quadrant
of the thorax.

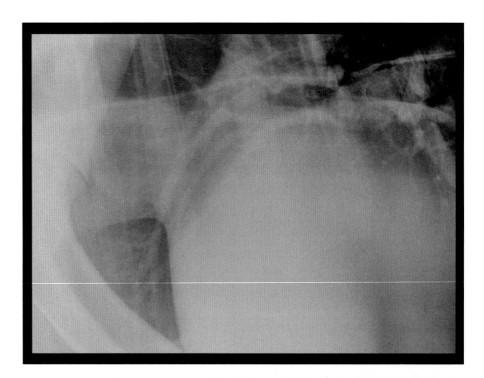

Figure 17.5
Radiographic anatomy of
the LL projection of the
cranioventral quadrant
of the thorax.

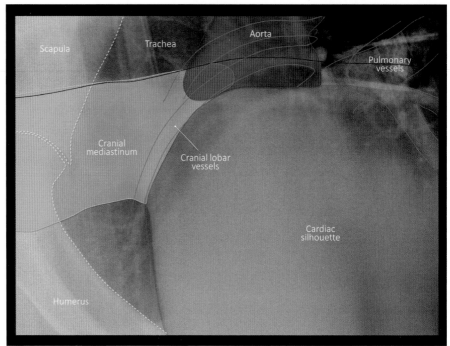

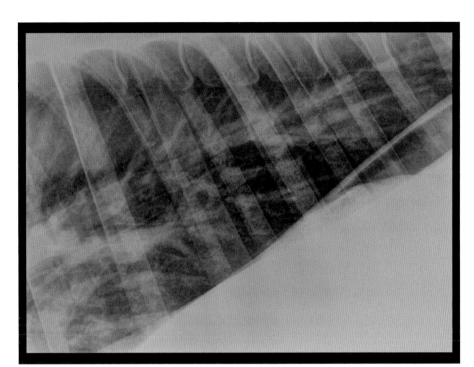

Figure 17.6
LL projection of the caudodorsal quadrant of the thorax.

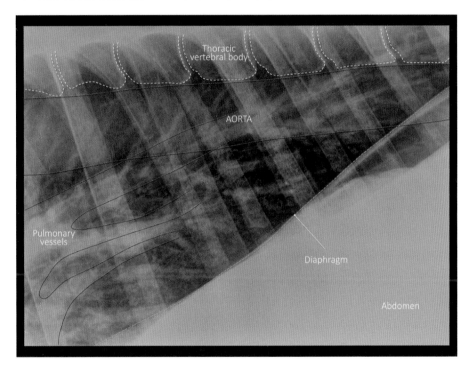

Figure 17.7
Radiographic anatomy of the LL projection of the caudodorsal quadrant of the thorax.

Figure 17.8
LL projection of the caudoventral quadrant of the thorax.

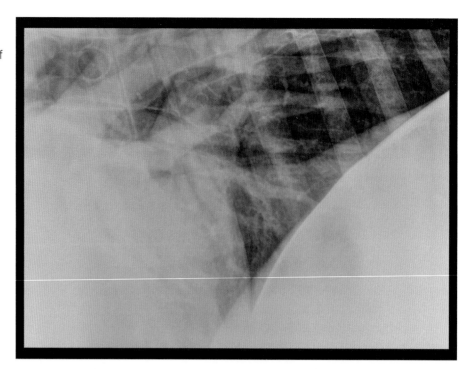

Figure 17.9
Radiographic anatomy of the LL projection of the caudoventral quadrant of the thorax.

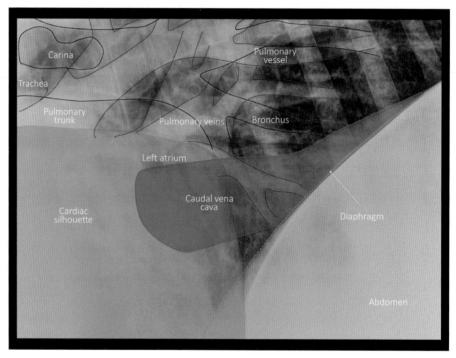

Laterolateral (LL) standing in foals (Figs 17.10–17.12)

1. Stand the foal square with all limbs equally weight-bearing, with the forelimbs slightly forward. Avoid any rotation or tilting of the body.
2. Place the plate on one side of the thorax in a vertical position in landscape orientation.
3. Indicate right/left (plate's side) with a marker.
4. Position the X-ray machine on the other side of the body.
5. Focus–film distance: 120 cm. If a grid is used, adjust the focus–film distance to the distance specified for the grid.
6. Use a horizontal X-ray beam, perpendicular to the long axis of the trunk.
7. Centre the X-ray beam in the middle third of the 8th intercostal space.
8. Collimate to the edge of the plate.
9. Exposure guide: 75 kVp, 30 mAs.

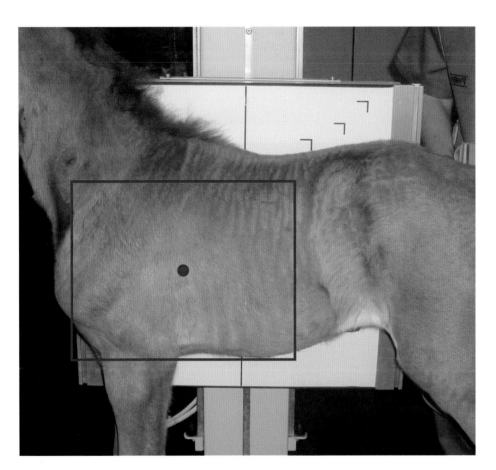

Figure 17.10 Positioning to obtain a LL view of the thorax in standing position in foals.

Figure 17.11
LL projection of the thorax in standing position in foals.

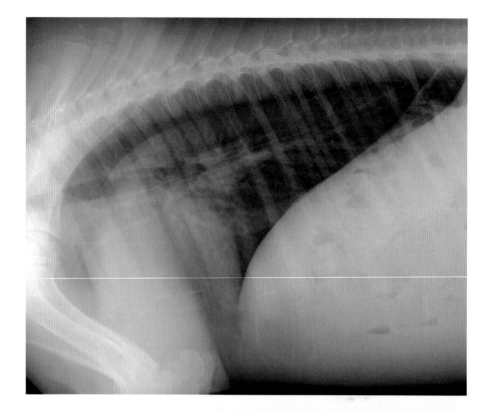

Figure 17.12
Radiographic anatomy of the LL projection of the thorax in standing position in foals.

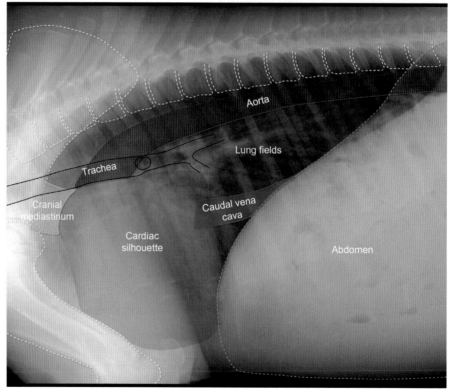

Laterolateral (LL) in lateral recumbency in foals (Figs 17.13–17.15)

1. Position the foal in lateral recumbency on a padded surface, keeping the neck parallel to the ground by supporting it and both forelimbs extended forward with gloved hands.
2. Place the plate under the thorax, in landscape orientation; a tunnel block will facilitate this.
3. Indicate right/left (plate's side) with a marker.
4. Position the X-ray machine above the foal.
5. Focus–film distance: 120 cm. If a grid is used, adjust the focus–film distance to the distance specified for the grid.
6. Use a vertical X-ray beam.
7. Centre the X-ray beam in the middle third of the 8th intercostal space.
8. Collimate to the edge of the plate.
9. Exposure guide: 75 kVp, 30 mAs.

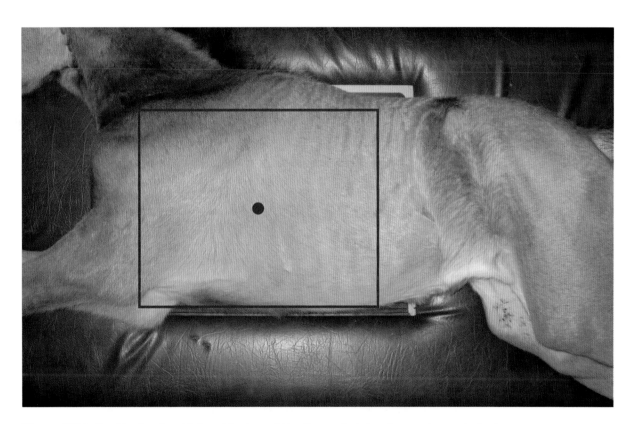

Figure 17.13 Positioning to obtain a LL view of the thorax in lateral recumbency in foals.

Figure 17.14
LL projection of
the thorax in lateral
recumbency in foals.

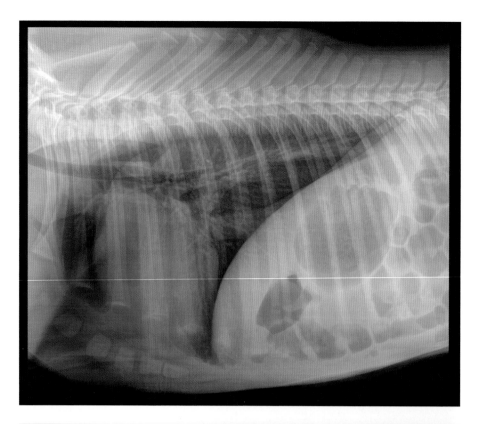

Figure 17.15
Radiographic anatomy
of the LL projection
of the thorax in lateral
recumbency in foals.

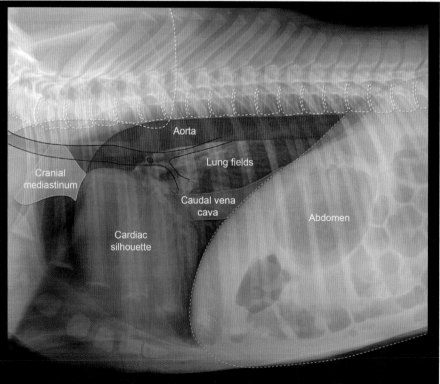

Ventrodorsal (VD) in foals
(Figs 17.16–17.18)

1. Position the foal in dorsal recumbency without rotation onto a padded surface, keeping the neck and both forelimbs extended forward and the hind limbs in a frog-leg position. Personnel involved in foal restraint must wear lead gloves.

2. Place the plate under the thorax, in portrait orientation along the long axis of the spine; a tunnel block will facilitate this.

3. Indicate right/left with a marker.

4. Position the X-ray machine above the foal.

5. Focus–film distance: 120 cm. If a grid is used, adjust the focus–film distance to the distance specified for the grid.

6. Use a vertical X-ray beam.

7. Centre the X-ray beam in the midline just caudal to the xiphoid process.

8. Collimate to the edge of the plate.

9. Exposure guide: 90 kVp, 40 mAs.

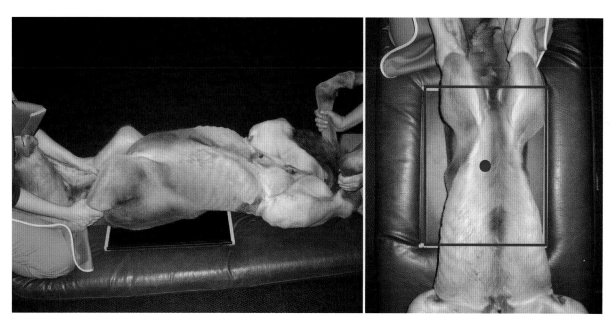

Figure 17.16 Positioning to obtain a VD view of the thorax in foals.

Figure 17.17
VD projection of the thorax in foals.

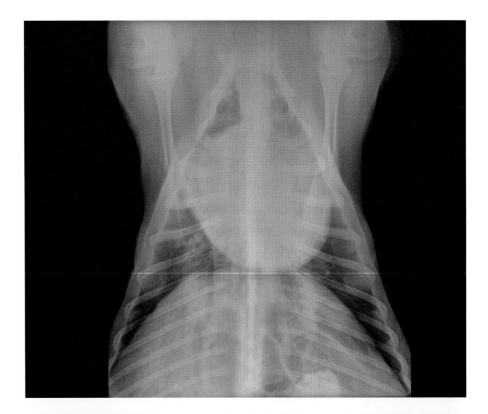

Figure 17.18
Radiographic anatomy of the VD projection of the thorax in foals.

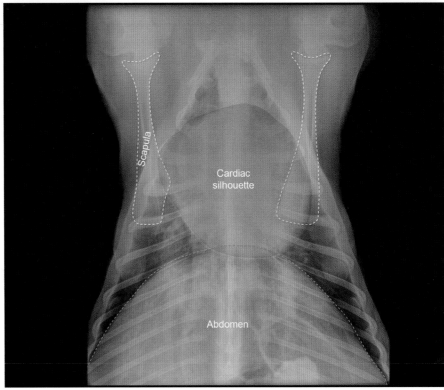

CHAPTER 18

Abdomen

Indications

Radiography of the abdomen is rarely performed in horses and limited to referral centres in adult, full-sized horses. Main indications for obtaining abdominal radiographs are:

- Investigation of chronic and recurrent colic episodes
- Suspected sand accumulation within the colon or presence of enteroliths
- Investigation of colic in foals, ponies and small horses
- Investigation of meconium impactions in foals.

Equipment

For a complete study of the thorax the following equipment is required:

- High-output X-ray generator
- Large plates (35 × 43 cm)
- Parallel grid, depending on the system used
- Mounted plate holder (ceiling- or wall-mounted)
- Radiation safety equipment: lead gowns and thyroid protectors.

Preparation

If necessary, brush or wash the area to reduce artefacts caused by dirt. Sedation of the patient is advised. Divide the abdomen according to the size of the plates so each view overlaps slightly.

Radiographic protocol

Radiographic protocol of the abdomen of an adult horse is composed of several overlapping laterolateral (LL) radiographs. The number of views depends on the suspected disease, with the most commonly evaluated area being the cranioventral aspect of the abdomen (Fig. 18.1). In foals and ponies, one or two views are enough (see Fig. 18.4).

Laterolateral (LL) in adult horses (Figs 18.1–18.3)

1. Stand the horse square with all limbs equally weight-bearing. Avoid any rotation or tilting of the body.
2. Place the plate on one side of the abdomen in a vertical position in landscape orientation.
3. Indicate right/left (plate's side) with a marker.
4. Position the X-ray machine on the other side of the body.
5. Focus–film distance: 120 cm. If a grid is used, adjust the focus–film distance to the distance specified for the grid.
6. Use a horizontal X-ray beam, perpendicular to the long axis of the trunk.
7. X-ray centring depends on the area to be evaluated.
8. Collimate to the edges of the plate.
9. Exposure guide: 150 kVp, 200 mAs.

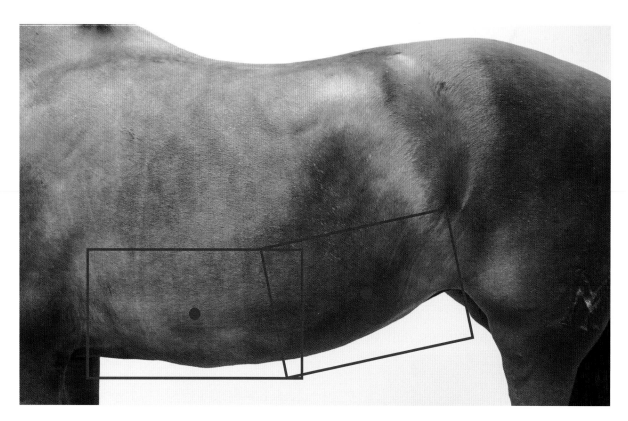

Figure 18.1 Positioning to obtain a LL view of the cranioventral aspect of the abdomen in adult horses.

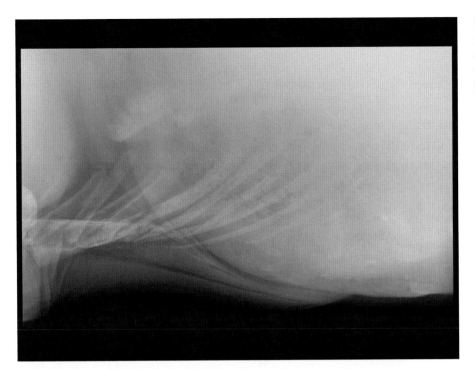

Figure 18.2
LL projection of the cranioventral aspect of the abdomen in adult horses.

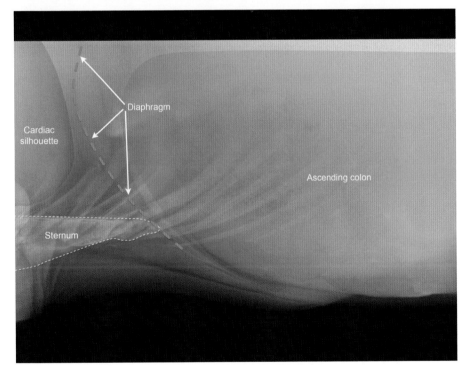

Figure 18.3
Radiographic anatomy of the LL projection of the cranioventral aspect of the abdomen in adult horses.

Laterolateral (LL) in foals (Figs 18.4 and 18.5)

1. Stand the foal square with all limbs equally weight-bearing. Avoid any rotation or tilting of the body.
2. Place the plate on one side of the abdomen in a vertical position in landscape orientation.
3. Indicate right/left (plate's side) with a marker.
4. Position the X-ray machine on the other side of the body.
5. Focus–film distance: 120 cm. If a grid is used, adjust the focus–film distance to the distance specified for the grid.
6. Use a horizontal X-ray beam, perpendicular to the long axis of the trunk.
7. X-ray centring depends on the size of the foal and the area to be evaluated. In newborn foals, centre in the middle third of the costal arch.
8. Collimate to the edges of the plate.
9. Exposure guide: 85 kVp, 50 mAs.

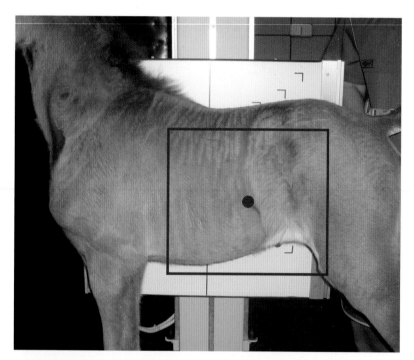

Figure 18.4 Positioning to obtain a LL view of the abdomen in foals.

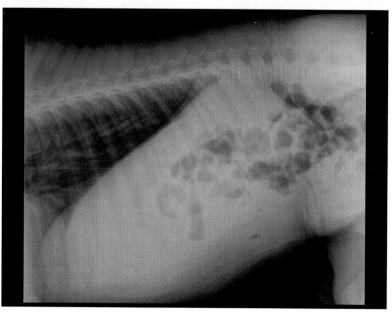

Figure 18.5 LL projection of the abdomen in foals.

INDEX